D1601615

LIVER TRANSPLANTATION

CLINICAL GASTROENTEROLOGY

George Y. Wu, Series Editor

LIVER
TRANSPLANTATION

CHALLENGING
CONTROVERSIES AND TOPICS

Edited by

GREGORY T. EVERSON, MD

University of Colorado,
Denver, USA

and

JAMES F. TROTTER, MD

University of Colorado,
Denver, USA

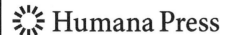 Humana Press

Editors
Gregory T. Everson, MD
University of Colorado
Health Sciences Center
Div. Gastroenterology & Hepatology
1635 N. Ursula, B-154
Aurora, CO 80045
greg.everson@uchsc.edu

James F. Trotter, MD
University of Colorado
Health Sciences Center
Div. Gastroenterology & Hepatology
1635 N. Ursula, B-154
Aurora, CO 80045
james.trotter@uchsc.edu

Series Editor
George Y. Wu, MD, PhD
University of Connecticut,
Farmington, Connecticut

ISBN: 978-1-58829-793-8   e-ISBN: 978-1-60327-028-1

Library of Congress Control Number: 2008938267

Printed on acid-free paper

9 8 7 6 5 4 3 2 1

springer.com

PREFACE

Liver Transplantation: Challenging Controversies and Topics grew out of a need I perceived within the fields of transplant hepatology and liver transplantation. Liver transplantation has rightly gained recognition as an established therapy for end-stage liver disease. Few would argue that liver transplantation is one of the few truly lifesaving and life-altering treatments within medicine and surgery. Not many realize that 20 years passed from the time of the first human liver transplantation in 1963 to its acceptance as therapy by the 1983 NIH Consensus Conference on Liver Transplantation. In 2008, 25 years will have passed since the 1983 NIH conference—a mere 25 years for a field that has provided patients hope, doctors options, and to some the "gift of life." Many issues in liver transplantation involve indications, patient selection, and outcomes after transplantation—these are standard topics, covered by textbooks of hepatology and transplantation. In contrast, the field of liver transplantation is young, evolving, dynamic, and issues and decisions are often controversial. Thus, Dr. Trotter and I, as well as our colleagues at the University of Colorado, felt that a text with a different focus was required, one that highlighted controversy and challenged dogma. Out of this perceived need emerged *Liver Transplantation: Challenging Controversies and Topics.*

To meet the transplant community's need for emerging information about liver transplantation, Dr. Larry Chan, Dr. Igal Kam, and I initiated the Controversies in Transplantation Conference. Many transplant physicians, transplant surgeons, and transplant professionals attend and participate in this meeting, and those who attend return! Why? Because the field is evolving, and many lessons remain to be learned by discussion, exchange of ideas, and challenge of dogma. As I saw interest grow and develop for our Controversies meeting, I realized that other media should be considered to maintain the discourse and challenge our colleagues and care providers. We next initiated the Young Investigators' Forum in Transplant Hepatology in order to embrace our junior and emerging colleagues in the process of defining issues, controversies, and challenging "fact" and dogma. Now, we have extended this concept to the written page. What began as a simple idea has turned into a long-term project that resulted in the publication of this first edition of *Liver Transplantation: Challenging Controversies and Topics.*

As we wrote and rewrote the text, we tried to create a useful set of chapters that would take the reader step by step through key areas of controversy in the field of liver transplantation. We tried to anticipate questions, define key issues, and provide options for resolving or approaching areas of uncertainty. The topics covered in this book impact our understanding and management of immunosuppression, viral hepatitis, nonalcoholic fatty liver disease, organ allocation, regional differences in rates of transplantation, and hepatocellular cancer. The contributors to this book are all actively practicing physicians and surgeons who deal with all the issues discussed in our text on a daily basis. The discussions are real and ongoing—often there may be no answer! In these pages, you will read the stories of active practitioners of transplant hepatology and liver transplantation from liver centers throughout the United States, Canada, and Australia who generously contributed their knowledge and experiences and encouraged us to complete the work.

Throughout the book we emphasize the need for thoughtful, well-controlled clinical and basic research of transplant hepatology and liver transplantation. We occasionally speculate on potential breakthroughs in immunology, virology, cell biology, surgery, and medicine that might influence or impact the future directions of these fields of medicine. My own career has been centered on investigation and research. I owe much of my clinical investigative activity to my late mentor, colleague, and friend, Dr. Fred Kern, Jr., my current colleague in transplantation, Dr. Igal Kam, and my many colleagues, nurses, coordinators, staff, and friends within the Division of Gastroenterology and Hepatology at the University of Colorado Health Sciences Center.

One last word: it is our hope that you will read, enjoy, and be stimulated by *Liver Transplantation: Challenging Controversies and Topics*. It is not meant to be a detailed reference guide; rather, the chapters and topics were selected to stimulate interest, identify topics requiring additional study, and promote discourse among transplant professionals. Read, enjoy, and be stimulated!

Gregory T. Everson, MD, FACP, FAGA
James F. Trotter, MD
February 2008

ACKNOWLEDGMENTS

We appreciate and gratefully acknowledge the hard-working, dedicated members of the Liver Team at the University of Colorado Health Sciences Center, who are always generous with their help and support: Lisa M. Forman, MD; James Burton, MD; Hugo Rosen, MD; Igal Kam, MD, Chief of Division of Transplant Surgery; Michael Wachs, MD; Thomas Bak, MD; Michael A. Zimmerman, MD; Susan Mandell, MD; Thomas Beresford, MD; Catherine Ray, RN, BSN, MA, Hepatology Nurse; Catherine Behnke, RN, Hepatology Nurse; Geri Martin, RN, Hepatology Nurse; Anne Shaver, RN, Hepatology Nurse; Andrea Petties, MA; Marge Frueh, Administrator of the Transplant Center; Jennifer DeSanto, RN, Research Coordinator; Andrea Herman, RN, Research Coordinator; Marlene Warren, RN, Research Coordinator; Laurie Fillar's, Research Coordinator; Tracy Steinberg, RN, MS, CCTC; Tim Brackett, RN; Mary McClure, RN; Michelle Miller, RN; Lana Schoch, RN; Michael Talamantes, MSSW, LCSW; and Lacye Cahill, MSSW, LCSW.

We also wish to further acknowledge the support of the staff at University Hospital and the University of Colorado Health Sciences Center in the care and management of our patients with liver disease and those patients and families confronted with liver transplantation. Special thanks to The Hep C Connection and to Hep C Connection support group members; the University Hospital Transplant Support Group; the Rocky Mountain Chapter of the American Liver Foundation; and all the patients with liver disease or liver transplantation across the country whose stories and problems have touched our lives and challenged us to do better!

Finally, this book would not have been possible without the efforts of our group of talented authors—we appreciate their honesty, critical thinking, and willingness to participate in this project.

Contents

Contributors

ROBERT S. BROWN, JR., MD, MPH • *The New York Presbyterian Hospital, Center for Liver Disease and Transplantation, New York, NY*

DAVID A. BRUNO, MD • *Transplantation Branch, National Institute of Diabetes, Digestive and Kidney Diseases, National Institutes of Health, Department of Health and Human Services, Bethesda, MD*

ANDREW M. CAMERON, MD, PHD • *Assistant Professor of Surgery, Division of Transplantation, The Johns Hopkins University School of Medicine, Baltimore, MD*

MICHAEL CHARLTON, MD • *Department of Gastroenterology and Hepatology, Mayo Clinic and Foundation, Rochester, MN*

MICHAEL B. FALLON, MD • *Liver Center, Division of Gastroenterology/Hepatology, Department of Medicine, University of Alabama at Birmingham, Birmingham, AL*

LISA M. FORMAN, MD • *Division of Gastroenterology and Hepatology, University of Colorado Health Sciences Center, Denver, CO*

RICHARD B. FREEMAN, JR., MD • *Division of Transplantation, Tufts University – New England Medical Center, Boston, MA*

QINCHUN FU, MD • *Shanghai Liver Disease Research Center, Shanghai, China*

R. MARK GHOBRIAL, MD, PHD • *Director, Liver Center; Chief, Liver Transplantation Surgery; Director, Immunobiology Research Center, The Methodist Hospital, Houston, Texas*

JADE D. JAMIAS, MD, FPCP, DPSG, DPSDE • *National Kidney and Transplant Institute, Quezon City, Philippines*

ALLAN D. KIRK, MD, PHD • *Transplantation Branch, National Institute of Diabetes, Digestive and Kidney Diseases, National Institutes of Health, Department of Health and Human Services, Bethesda, MD*

NORMAN M. KNETEMAN, MD, MSC, MSM • *Department of Surgery, Section of Hepatobiliary, Pancreatic and Transplant Surgery University of Alberta, Edmonton, Canada*

ANDREW L. MASON, MB, BS • *Department of Medicine, Division of Gastroenterology, University of Alberta, Edmonton, Alberta, Canada*

GEOFFREY MCCAUGHAN, MBBS, MD, FRACP, PHD • *AW Morrow Gastroenterology and Liver Centre, Royal Prince Alfred Hospital, Camperdown, New South Wales, Australia*

DAVID T. PALMA, MD • *Liver Center, Division of Gastroenterology/Hepatology, Department of Medicine, University of Alabama at Birmingham, Birmingham, AL*

MARIO G. PESSOA • *Division of Gastroenterology, University of California, San Francisco, San Francisco, CA, Sao Paulo, Brazil*

JOHN F. RENZ, MD, PHD • *Department of Surgery, Center for Liver Disease and Transplantation, The New York Presbyterian Hospital, New York, NY*

NICHOLAS SHACKEL, MBBS, MD, FRACP, PHD • *AW Morrow Gastroenterology and Liver Centre, Royal Prince Alfred Hospital, Camperdown, New South Wales, Australia*

SIMONE STRASSER, MBBS, MD, FRACP • *AW Morrow Gastroenterology and Liver Centre, Royal Prince Alfred Hospital, Camperdown, New South Wales, Australia*

NORAH A. TERRAULT, MD, MPH • *Division of Gastroenterology, University of California, San Francisco, San Francisco, CA*

CHRISTIAN TOSO • *Department of Surgery, Section of Hepatobiliary, Pancreatic and Transplant Surgery, University of Alberta, Edmonton, Alberta, Canada*

MICHAEL A. ZIMMERMAN, MD • *Assistant Professor of Surgery, University of Colorado Health Sciences Center, Division of Transplant Surgery, Denver, CO*

1

Tolerance in Liver Transplantation
Just a Promise or an Evolving Reality?

David A. Bruno, MD
and Allan D. Kirk, MD, PhD

CONTENTS

INTRODUCTION
DEFINING THE CHALLENGES
UNIQUE ASPECTS OF THE LIVER
    INFLUENCING IMMUNE OUTCOME
CLINICAL TOLERANCE
CONCLUSIONS
REFERENCES

Abstract

In recent years, a variety of immunosuppressive (IS) agents has emerged. The best application and combination of these new agents along with traditional immunosuppressive agents present challenges and opportunities to transplant physicians. Two anti-IL2 receptor monoclonal antibodies are currently available for clinical use: daclizumab (Zenapax, Roche) and basiliximab (Simulect, Novartis). Both bind to the alpha subunit of the IL-2 receptor (CD-25), which is expressed on activated, but not resting, lymphocytes. These

From: *Clinical Gastroenterology: Liver Transplantation: Challenging
Controversies and Topics*
Edited by: G. T. Everson and J. F. Trotter, DOI: 10.1007/978-1-60327-028-1_1,
© Humana Press, Totowa, NJ

drugs are the most commonly used induction agents in the United States. Campath-1H (C-1H) or alemtuzumab (Ilex Pharmacenticals) has been used in a limited fashion in liver transplantation recipients with mixed results. The role of sirolimus in liver transplantation remains controversial. However, this agent may offer specific advantages in patients with hepatocellular carcinoma or renal dysfunction. Because hepatitis C is the most common indication for liver transplantation, the application of immunosuppression in these patients is important. However, the best regimen for these patients remains controversial. The role of new immunosuppressive drugs including FTY720, FK778, and LEA29Y offers the promise for better immunosuppression for future liver transplantation recipients.

Key Words: Immunosuppression; Interleukin receptor antagonist; Campath; Sirolimus; Hepatitis C; Hepatocellular carcinoma

INTRODUCTION

In humans, all vascularized allografts undergo immune-mediated rejection unless some modification is made to the recipient's immune system. There has not been a single case report of an immunocompetent human accepting any allograft without some intercurrent immunologically consequential therapy or illness. Thus, we must assume that the first rule for human liver transplantation is that allografts are rejected.

The first rule of transplantation not withstanding, it has been established that liver allografts are less likely to be lost to rejection than other solid organs (1–4). Similarly, clinicians have empirically determined that excellent survival rates can be achieved with less immunosuppressive therapy compared to other organs (5). As such, the liver has been increasingly described as "tolerogenic," suggesting that the liver possesses unique qualities that quell immune rejection. Indeed, the clinical approach to liver transplantation has long been shaped by the comparative ease with which immunosuppression can be eliminated or reduced substantially in humans (6–9). When complete immunosuppressive elimination has been achieved, it has been described as "spontaneous" tolerance, but in reality, all accepted grafts have been achieved through significant immune manipulation or an initial episode of rejection and, in controlled analysis, are closely related to MHC match (10). Thus, while it appears that the liver is more easily guided into a situation of immune equilibrium, the bridge to tolerance is not passively traversed.

Several lines of objective evidence illustrating the liver's unique immune qualities speak to its ability to be tolerated more readily than other vascular allografts. The Chase–Sulzberger effect, or the tolerance to oral antigens, has long been recognized, reproduced experimentally, and shown to be dependent on enterohepatic blood flow (11–15). Similarly, tolerance has been induced to antigens introduced via the portal circulation (16). Nonhepatic allograft survival has also been reported to be improved when a liver allograft is included, suggesting a dominant and systemic effect (2, 17–21). Most importantly, there may be an increased rate of successful immunosuppressive weaning in recipients of liver transplants compared to other vascularized organs (6–9). Can these effects be codified and harnessed for clinical purposes? Given the exceptionally good results of transplantation under current immunosuppressive regimens, is the likelihood of tolerance substantial and consistent enough to make it a clinically important strategy? Finally, is tolerance a durable state, or instead is it a metastable condition destined to fail at some predictable rate? This chapter will summarize the unique properties of the liver that relate to its immunological behavior and outline the biological properties that likely influence the need for immunosuppression following allogeneic liver transplantation. Specific attention will be given to the limitations of tolerance as a modern clinical strategy.

DEFINING THE CHALLENGES

Several very basic issues are paramount to understanding the liver's unique immune properties. Most critical is the recognition that tolerance, immunosuppression, and rejection are broad clinical terms that describe the aggregate result of many competing and complementary processes. None of these terms has a biological meaning that suggests mechanisms of action. One can be immunosuppressed via many mechanisms and still not be tolerant. Similarly, rejection can result from immunosuppression (e.g., suppressed regulation), and tolerance from immune activation (activation-induced cell death). Thus, the first requirement for a discussion of tolerance is to dispense with broad generalities and define the biology involved.

As clinicians, we may see immunosuppression, tolerance, and rejection as binary absolutes and, in doing so, we mistake a phenotype of tolerance for a robust condition when it is but a passing period of immune quiescence or endogenous immunoincompetence. It is more appropriate to recognize all of the mechanisms influencing rejection or acceptance as spectral, operating via relative degrees of influence, not presence or absence. As such, each patient presents as a mosaic of genetic predispositions, environmental and pharmacological influences, organ characteristics (e.g., regenerative ability, size), and prior and future immune experiences that together produce a clinical immune phenotype. Tolerance can result via a combination of factors and, given the complexity of the factors involved, almost certainly is not the result of any single treatment or approach. Thus, it would be erroneous to postulate that all patients in receipt of any liver would meet the criteria for immunosuppressive withdrawal. As such, a critical question is whether it is possible to prospectively determine who can become tolerant, particularly when the consequences of failure are not benign (22).

A second basic concern is one of timing. As adaptive immunity is, by definition, adaptive, defining its behavior at any point in time will not necessarily predict future behavior. It is now clear that environmental exposures markedly alter the active T cell repertoire (23). Given that we cannot predict future infections or antigens that one might encounter, a significant barrier may be determining an individual's future alloresponsiveness. Indeed, the concept of an immune system that is both fully competent and forever incapable of mediating a response to novel antigens is flawed. Perhaps the most startling illustration of this is liver rejection in the native liver, or autoimmune hepatitis. Although we have established through the first rule that alloimmunity is a probable, if not inevitable, event, and by clinical observation that autoimmunity is a possible albeit improbable event—both do indeed occur. In light of this, it must be recognized that the achievement of tolerance in transplantation is unlikely to exceed that of the population to their native organs. With this in mind, we must recognize at the outset that the interaction among immune system, environment, host, and allograft likely prevents any generalized therapeutic maneuver that will lead to universal tolerance.

The tie that binds both of these concepts is one of complexity. Accordingly, the science of complex systems is useful in understanding how to approach the topic of tolerance in any organ system. Formalized by Lorenz and subsequently by Yorke, the chaos theory (24, 25) provides a framework in which to assess complex dynamic systems. In general, the reliability of forecasts in dynamical systems deteriorates exponentially over time due to a sensitive dependence on a complete, but unfortunately unachievable, characterization of the conditions governing the process. Forecasts can be improved by limiting the number of variables in a system, in effect making it less complex, but biology does not offer this luxury. Although the specifics are beyond the scope of this chapter, in general, when there are multiple competing and complementary factors influencing an outcome, we will forever be forced to assess outcomes based on probability rather than certainty, and our ability to ascertain probability will worsen as we try to predict farther into the future. In situations like these, the common endpoint tends to gravitate back to fundamental conditions; for allografts, this is rejection. Thus, most patients, if immunocompetent, will eventually reject. Success will therefore be measured by the rate and consequences of rejection relative to the rate of the adverse effects of immunosuppressants.

Based on these principles, tolerance, defined as acceptable graft function without medications, will only be successful to the extent that it generates aggregate outcomes that exceed those associated with immunosuppression. If many, perhaps all, liver transplant recipients can be weaned to lower doses of immunosuppressive agents, and suffer fewer side effects of chronic immunosuppression relative to other organ recipients, then the bar for tolerance must be set even higher. Furthermore, it will need to be predictable and analyzed on an intent-to-treat basis. For example, a 30% tolerance rate that evokes a 70% rejection rate will likely not be an acceptable clinical standard. The quest for tolerance in the liver, and in all organs, must be carried out using specific measures of success weighed against the inevitable consequences of failure.

UNIQUE ASPECTS OF THE LIVER INFLUENCING IMMUNE OUTCOME

The unique nature of hepatic immunity has long been a subject of interest in the laboratory and the clinic (26–28). As is often the case, observations in the clinic have led to answers in the lab. What makes the liver pro-tolerant? What unique combinations of factors act to shift the balance in the liver toward regulation?

In order to establish reasonable rules for identifying tolerance in liver recipients, it is important to understand the objective considerations controlling hepatic immunity. All cellular immune responses, including those to liver allografts, have basic similarities that should be considered in assessing the likely outcome. They include the precursor frequency of responding cells relative to the target population, fundamental target susceptibility, and an environment that either supports or inhibits the response. Relative to other organs, all of these factors in the liver favor tolerance.

While the T cell precursor frequency of alloantigens expressed by the liver is no different than for similar alloantigens on other organs, it is clearly lower relative to the target cell population. The ratio of the size of the liver to the allospecific T cell repertoire is massive; thus, each liver cell begins with a statistical advantage—a lower effector-to-target ratio compared to other organs. While this may be a simplistic assertion, it would be difficult to argue the converse.

Organ susceptibility also favors the liver relative to other organs. A liver's unique regenerative capacity exceeds that of other parenchymal organs. As such, any degree of injury is likely to be borne with greater resilience by the liver. All immune responses are subject to balanced rates of destruction versus repair. In the case of the liver, relatively more destruction is required to achieve a given phenotype of injury. The subject of hepatic regeneration has recently gained momentum and is clearly an important aspect of the liver's recovery from injury (29). Regeneration does not speak directly to immune tolerance, but it most certainly alters the clinical perception that a tolerant phenotype exists.

While precursor frequency and regeneration likely alter our perception of the degree and pace of rejection, many other aspects of the liver's unique vascular environment form the basis for true pro-tolerant behavior. This is typically framed in relation to the liver's physiological role in maintaining immune homeostasis despite continuous antigen exposure via the portal circulation. Whereas epithelial organs (skin, gut, lung, and kidney) act as a barrier, preventing entry of environmental pathogens, the liver is specifically concerned with making use of antigenic molecules for metabolic processing. The liver must also discriminate between pathogens and antigens from symbiotic organisms critical to host survival such as gut flora that at times enter the portal circulation. This discriminatory role is facilitated through several unique anatomical and cellular properties of the liver.

Hepatic afferent blood flow is derived from both the hepatic artery and the portal vein. Arterial blood and portal venous blood mix in unique sinusoids and transit from portal tracts to the central veins (see Fig. 1) (27, 30–32). These sinusoids are covered by specialized endothelial cells known as liver sinusoidal endothelial cells (LSECs) (26, 28). Whereas most endothelia are free of the molecules facilitating effective antigen presentation, like the costimulatory molecules CD80 and CD86, and are poor antigen presenting cells (APCs), LSECs constitutively express these molecules and are known to function as APCs. Interestingly, intrahepatic antigen presentation by LSECs typically evokes an anergic or regulatory state in the responding T cells, suggesting a default response favoring tolerance (33, 34). This is in contrast to the typical effector response evoked when antigen is presented in the extrahepatic secondary lymphoid tissue (35). Such a stance is easily reconciled with the physiological role of the liver, to utilize antigens for metabolic purposes, and its placement behind a potent barrier organ, the gut.

The unique immune characteristics of the liver are clearly related to the liver's unique cellular architecture. Specifically, the liver sinusoids create a small-diameter system that induces slow velocity flow and periodic stasis. This facilitates close contact between the peripheral

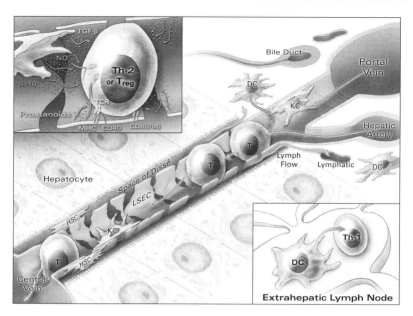

Fig. 1. Sinusoids anatomically support slow or static flow as blood flows from the portal vein and hepatic artery toward the central vein. Kupffer cells, LSECs, and dendritic cells incorporate antigen for presentation. Antigen engagement in the sinusoids (above left) promotes a nonaggressive immune response due to multiple soluble factors including IL-10, NO, and TGF-β. In contrast, hepatic DCs (below right) that migrate out of the sinusoids via lymphatics present antigen to extrahepatic lymph nodes and promote a Th1 or effector response.

blood (30% of which circulates through the liver every minute) and specialized LSECs (36). These cells line the liver sinusoid walls and serve as a selective barrier for macromolecules and cells, controlling direct contact between hepatocytes and blood elements. These are distinct from Kupffer cells, which are phagocytic cells that patrol the sinusoids but do not have direct contact with hepatocytes. While Kupffer cells provide the general phagocytic function of sinusoidal debris and are thought to play a major role in endotoxin clearance and intact microorganism clearance, LSECs specifically deliver macromolecules to the hepatocytes and, as such, need to present these potential antigens without immune activation. In addition to expressing critical costimulatory and adhesion molecules required for effective antigen presentation, LSECs also express the mannose receptor and scavenger receptors used in phagocytosis on prokaryotic organisms (37, 38).

There is accumulating evidence that cells activated by LSECs preferentially develop an anergic or regulatory function with a predominantly Th-2 phenotype (39). Teleologically, lymphocytes primed in the liver are more likely to present antigen that is of some nutritional benefit, or related to symbiotic flora, whereas antigen initially encountered in peripheral lymph nodes may be more likely to be pathogenic. The distinction needs only be based on generalities and evoke a weak preference to influence the evolution of an immune response. Under more vigorous inflammatory conditions, LSECs are capable of inducing a protective response. However, it is clear that T cell activation within the hepatic parenchyma is typically detrimental (40). Indeed, when polyclonal T cell activation is induced in the liver experimentally, severe T cell-mediated parenchymal damage follows, indicating that, in general, activated T cells are unwelcome in the hepatic microenvironment.

The mechanisms by which LSECs and Kupffer cells contain T cell reactivity are currently the subject of investigation. However, both cell types constitutively support a paracrine milieu that is consistent with immune regulation. Under general conditions with physiological doses of portal endotoxin, Kupffer cells express IL-10, TGF-β, nitric oxide, and prostanoids that limit T cell reactivity and favor a nonaggressive immune response (41). Similarly, LSECs constitutively express prostanoids, which also limit the antigen presentation activity of the LSECs and promote an immunologically quiescent posture (42). Allogeneic LSECs could potentially prevent activation of allospecific T cells and facilitate the direct neutering of alloreactive T cells.

The unique properties of LSEC and Kupffer cells may also lead to donor-specific T cell depletion. It also appears that Kupffer cells and LSECs can induce apoptosis of activated T cells (39, 43, 44). This may be a mechanism by which portal venous antigen injection leads to antigen-specific tolerance. After liver transplantation, donor antigen, in the form of major histocompatibility complex class I molecules, is present in great quantities (45). This donor antigen is potentially taken up by the LSECs and presented in a context that avoids T cell activation (46). Thus, allospecific T cells that encounter antigen in the LSEC environment undergo apoptosis, facilitating a reduction in precursor frequency. Apoptotic cells are then preferentially trapped in the liver through receptor-mediated processes.

The unique separation of blood from the hepatic parenchyma introduces some element of ignorance in hepatic tolerance. It has been experimentally shown that antigens expressed solely on the hepatic parenchyma cannot be cleared by antigen-specific T cells (43). This is a fundamental problem in hepatitis. Hepatotropism of viruses is not explained by receptor-mediated targeting of hepatocytes. Rather, experimental models of hepatitis such as the duck HBV model show that even when the viral receptor is ubiquitously expressed, only hepatocytes become infected (47, 48). This suggests that the virus preferentially infects liver cells through some means of immune evasion unique to the liver either by Trojan horse entry via the LSEC or through LSEC-mediated tolerance in the hepatic environment. Ignorance prevents immune responses once inside the cell, and subsequent processed antigen presentation via LSECs tends to favor tolerance in the absence of concomitant inflammation or cell lysis.

Even though antigen is released and available for uptake and presentation by nonhepatocytes, it is unlikely to be advantageous to do so. Nonlytic infections are not in and of themselves detrimental: The immune response to them is. Thus, the LSEC may play an important role in quelling nonadvantageous immunity favoring anergy and establishment of a carrier state. Furthermore, antigen uptake is receptor-mediated particularly via innate pattern recognition receptors such as the mannose receptors.

Several other cell types shape intrahepatic immune responses. The liver is rich in resident dendritic cells (DCs). These cells are also thought to have unique tendencies to induce tolerance to presented antigens. Hepatic DCs are likely influenced by the IL-10 and TGF-β constitutively expressed by Kupffer cells and LSECs, and mediate some of their effects through T cells expressing CD152 and PD-1 (49–51). Hepatic DCs are known to migrate to extrahepatic sites where they may be capable of influencing systemic immune responses. Indeed, it is this migration that has featured prominently in the clinical hepatic tolerance literature discussed ahead (4, 52, 53). The liver is also rich in NK T cells, a cell population that has been suggested to mediate pro-tolerant effects (54).

Unique Toll-like receptor expression on hepatic DCs also helps to establish a biological explanation for the apparent pro-tolerant posture of hepatic DCs. Liver DCs have reduced expression of TLR4 compared to splenic DCs, correlating with a reduced ability of the LPS-stimulated liver DCs to activate T cells to express interferon-γ (55). Hepatic DCs were shown to markedly differ functionally and phenotypically with splenic DCs, with hepatic DCs showing a bias toward tolerance.

The reach of intrahepatic tolerance mechanisms may indeed spread to extrahepatic sites. It has been shown that LSEC antigen presentation evokes a regulatory T cell phenotype (33, 34, 56). T cells expressing CD4, CD25, and CD152 derived from LSEC exposure can be used to transfer a tolerant phenotype from one experimental animal to another and would presumably be able to inhibit peripheral immune responses within the same animal. Thus, allospecific regulation could be derived from recipient T cells encountering alloantigen directly within the sinusoids. Similarly, there has been speculation that LSECs are also involved in the regulation of general systemic inflammation. There are almost no situations where systemic activation of the immune system is advantageous. In general, this leads to shock and death. Thus, when antigen is systemically disseminated, it will be presented by LSECs and lead to one of the mechanisms of immune attenuation listed above. Thus, LSECs may prevent systemic cellular effects of trauma as well as hepatocyte damage.

Finally, in addition to physiological mechanisms promoting tolerance, the pathology of liver failure may also contribute to a generally hyporesponsive state. Hepatic failure may attenuate the initial response to an allograft through depletion of complement and clotting cascade factors known to serve as immune adjuvants and opsonins. Similarly, hypersplenism resulting from portal hypertension frequently leads to thrombocytopenia, and platelets are increasingly being recognized as strong inducers of rejection. Platelet-derived CD154 has been shown to induce rejection independent of cell-bound sources of this important costimulatory molecule (57).

Most of these pro-tolerant mechanisms are balanced by pro-inflammatory potential. Thus, the liver favors tolerance but is not locked into it. As with most biological processes, the liver falls along a spectrum that can be perturbed by inflammation. The space between the LSECs and the hepatocytes is the space of Disse. There is no basement membrane; lymphocytes and plasma that extravasates into the space of Disse become lymph, which drains to extrahepatic nodes. Thus, factors that are not effectively processed intrahepatically are certainly available for presentation in the nodes; presumably, this provides stimulation competing with the intrahepatic processes for tolerance.

CLINICAL TOLERANCE

It is important to distinguish absolute mechanisms from relative mechanisms. Absolute mechanisms leave the individual incapable of rejection; to date, there are no clinically applicable absolutes in allospecific tolerance. Relative mechanisms improve the likelihood of a salutary outcome. They alter a rate or a likelihood of rejection, but their value must be compared to the risks associated with immunosuppressive withdrawal. Given the first rule of transplants, "organs reject," all mechanisms discussed will be clinically useful only to the extent that they balance the clinical consequences of immunosuppression. The theory of tolerance should not be evoked to counter the first rule unless there is a compelling side effect profile that is being addressed. Even the robust

Medawarian tolerance that has defined our quest since its inception was only a 60% endeavor (3 of 5 mice) when originally described (58). Thus, clinical application of any of the above mechanisms becomes a practical matter of reproducibility and predictability.

The benefits of tolerance seem clear: organ replacement without the burden of chronic maintenance immunosuppression. However, those benefits may have differential applicability to the diverse diseases treated with transplantation. For example, the preservation of protective viral immunity may greatly improve the outcome of patients with viral hepatitis, while patients with autoimmune hepatitis may suffer greater disease recurrence without immune suppression. Similarly, the benefits of tolerance must be viewed in the light of their consistent practical attainability and durability. As such, the step from theory to practice must be taken with objectivity and some element of predictability. Regardless, patient outcome gauged against the current norm will be the measure of success, not the elimination of immunosuppression. At present, there are no clinical data prospectively evaluating outcome on an intent-to-treat basis.

There are a growing number of small reports investigating immunosuppressive withdrawal suggesting that many, but not most, liver transplant patients can be withdrawn from immunosuppression. Ramos et al., reporting from the Pittsburgh experience, first detailed the prospective withdrawal from immunosuppression in selected liver recipients (9). This experience was expanded two years later by Mazariegos et al. (59). These reports showed that in carefully selected individuals who were rejection-free by prospective biopsy and at least two years' posttransplant, sustained freedom from immunosuppressive drugs was achievable in 18 of 95 patients (19%). Interestingly, 2 of 13 patients with autoimmune primary biliary cirrhosis experienced recurrent disease during the study, and one long-term patient off all immunosuppression lost his liver from recurrent hepatitis C virus. This report exhibits the full spectrum of effects, both salutary and adverse, of drug withdrawal.

Devlin et al. reported on the Kings College experience of 18 liver recipients selected for withdrawal to address documented immunosuppressive complications after at least five years of stable graft function (60). Five patients (28%) were successfully weaned from all immunosuppression. Again, this report was remarkable for postwean flares in autoimmunity. Additionally, most patients had perturbations in previously stable hepatic transaminases, suggesting that a satisfactory outcome was the result of actively quelled alloimmunity and not from passive acceptance of the graft. No factor predicted success, including disease status, HLA mismatch, or chimerism. Furthermore, there was no indication that the patient's outcome was improved by the withdrawal. Complications attributed to immunosuppression, including hypertension, were not reported to be resolved postwithdrawal.

Girlanda et al. recently followed up on the Kings experience (61). Of the original 18 patients in which weaning was attempted, only the group of four patients who were unsuccessfully weaned and remained on all immunosuppression remained as a group alive and well. Of the five patients who were weaned from all immunosuppression and reported as stable in the original paper, three had returned to immunosuppression, one of whom required retransplantation, revising the actual rate of stable withdrawal to 11%. This again emphasizes that success cannot be defined by removal of immunosuppression, but rather will depend on patient outcome.

Considerable interest has been directed toward the pediatric liver transplant population, with the hypothesis that younger immune systems are more adaptive and perhaps more apt to foster tolerance. Furthermore, with live donor liver transplantation from parents, the degree of HLA match could be expected to facilitate immunosuppressive withdrawal. Indeed, a third of the patients reported in the Pittsburgh experience were children. It is interesting to point out that this suggests that the recipient immune response is the deciding factor and not so much the immune characteristics of the donor liver.

Takatsuki et al. reported on a withdrawal trial involving 63 pediatric recipients of live donor liver segments (7), a series that was updated to 115 patients (62). Patients were stratified based on protocol weaning (patients with more than two years of stable, rejection-free survival; $n = 67$) and nonprotocol weaning (patients weaned due to complications or noncompliance). Forty-two percent of patients were weaned off all immunosuppression. No deaths or graft losses were attributable to weaning. Again, there were no characteristics that predicted success. In fact, weaning was not more successful if performed under protocol conditions compared to nonprotocol conditions. As a recent follow-up, Ueda et al. have reported that patients deemed tolerant on clinical grounds can be shown by protocol biopsy to have ongoing ductal injury (63). Thus, as with other organs, subclinical rejection can occur, highlighting the importance of careful scrutiny in defining patient outcome. Indeed, tolerance should not be defined as slow rejection or failure to look for rejection.

Pons et al. studied nine stable allograft recipients more than two years posttransplant who underwent weaning (64). Three were successfully weaned. In five of these patients, a donor recipient sex discrepancy allowed the investigators to ask the specific question of whether endothelial cell chimerism on protocol biopsy—mixing of donor and recipient origin endothelial cells within the graft—was predictive of successful weaning. Chimerism did not appear to correlate with success.

More recently, Eason et al. reported on a prospective trial involving 18 patients who were stable and rejection-free at least six months posttransplant on monotherapy tacrolimus (22). Of these, only one was successfully weaned, and 11 experienced rejection, a markedly worse result that other reports in the literature. Of note is that three were weaned but were returned to immunosuppression for modest elevations in transaminases. This study suggests two possibilities: first, that six months is too early to begin immunosuppressive withdrawal; second, that the return to immunosuppression was perhaps premature, as other studies have consistently reported hypertransaminasemia that resolved without sequelae.

In 2006, Tisone et al. described a series of 34 adult (mean age: 62 ± 6 years) patients transplanted due to hepatitis C virus in whom weaning was attempted specifically to prevent viral progression (6). This study was supported by protocol biopsies. Eight patients (23%) were successfully weaned, a number remarkably similar to most other reports. All patients were at least one year posttransplant, and those successfully weaned were at least two years posttransplant. Several important observations were made regarding factors correlating with success. First, the freedom from immunosuppression had a measurable impact on hepatic fibrosis, with five weaning-tolerant patients showing improvement in the grading of the disease and none experiencing worsening. This contrasted to the weaning-intolerant group, in whom 42% of patients worsened histologically. Second, an intriguing statistically significant correlation was found between a low cyclosporine level in the first week after transplant and successful weaning. This provides suggestive validation of the Window of Functional Immune Engagement (WOFIE) theory proposed by Calne in his studies of *prope* tolerance (65). Thus, in this latter report, there is some evidence that weaning may improve outcome in selected disease states and that immune management early may impact subsequent immune behavior.

CONCLUSIONS

Taken together, the experimental and clinical data have allowed several generalizations to be formed to help guide future study. Viewed theoretically, the liver has clear anatomical, teleological, and immunological properties that support its status as immunologically unique, and there are credible scenarios related to specialized antigen presentation and cell migration that could, and likely do, produce both intrahepatic and systemic immune attenuation. Experimentally, tolerance can reproducibly be achieved using a variety of methods that are typically not successful with other organs. Thus, there is ample reason to view the liver as different and strive to exploit its differences to the benefit of transplant recipients.

Balanced against these factors are several clinical caveats. At present, immunosuppressive weaning applies only to carefully selected and monitored patients, likely only after two years of graft stability. Even with careful selection, success is not predictable, nor is it typical. The first rule still usually applies: Allografts are rejected. Importantly, attempts to achieve clinical tolerance have yet to be demonstrated as beneficial. As we cannot identify tolerance prospectively, intent-to-treat trials with long-term follow-up supported by protocol biopsies will be required, and these trials must be designed to objectively measure the potential benefits and pitfalls of drug withdrawal. Multicenter efforts should now be used, as there are sufficient single-center trials justifying broader study. Above all, we must define success based on patient outcome, not the amount of medication involved.

Acknowledgments

This manuscript was supported by the Intramural Research Program of the National Institute of Diabetes and Digestive and Kidney Diseases, National Institutes of Health, Department of Health and Human Services.

REFERENCES

1. Calne RY, Sells RA, Pena JR, Ashby BS, Herbertson BM, Millard PR, et al. Toleragenic effects of porcine liver allografts. *Br J Surg* 1969; 56(9):692–3.
2. Kamada N, Davies HS, Roser B. Reversal of transplantation immunity by liver grafting. *Nature* 1981; 292(5826):840–2.
3. Kamada N, Davies HS, Wight D, Culank L, Roser B. Liver transplantation in the rat. Biochemical and histological evidence of complete tolerance induction in non-rejector strains. *Transplantation* 1983; 35(4):304–11.
4. Starzl TE, Demetris AJ, Murase N, Ildstad S, Ricordi C, Trucco M. Cell migration, chimerism, and graft acceptance. *Lancet* 1992; 339(8809):1579–82.
5. Shapiro R, Young JB, Milford EL, Trotter JF, Bustami RT, Leichtman AB. Immunosuppression: Evolution in practice and trends, 1993–2003. *Am J Transpl* 2005; 5(4 Pt 2):874–86.
6. Tisone G, Orlando G, Cardillo A, Palmieri G, Manzia TM, Baiocchi L, et al. Complete weaning off immunosuppression in HCV liver transplant recipients is feasible and favourably impacts on the progression of disease recurrence. *J Hepatol* 2006; 44(4): 702–9.

7. Takatsuki M, Uemoto S, Inomata Y, Egawa H, Kiuchi T, Fujita S, et al. Weaning of immunosuppression in living donor liver transplant recipients. *Transplantation* 2001; 72(3):449–54.

8. Mazariegos GV, Reyes J, Marino IR, Demetris AJ, Flynn B, Irish W, et al. Weaning of immunosuppression in liver transplant recipients. *Transplantation* 1997; 63(2):243–9.

9. Ramos HC, Reyes J, Abu-Elmagd K, Zeevi A, Reinsmoen N, Tzakis A, et al. Weaning of immunosuppression in long-term liver transplant recipients. *Transplantation* 1995; 59(2):212–7.

10. Flye MW, Pennington L, Kirkman R, Weber B, Sindelar W, Sachs DH. Spontaneous acceptance or rejection of orthotopic liver transplants in outbred and partially inbred miniature swine. *Transplantation* 1999; 68(5):599–607.

11. Chase MW. Inhibition of experimental drug allergy by prior feeding of the sensitizing agent. *Proc Soc Exp Biol Med* 1946; 61:2579.

12. Sulzberger MB. Hypersensitiveness to neoarsphenamine in guinea-pigs: Experiments in prevention and in desensitization. *Arch Derm Syph* 1929; 20:669–81.

13. Ilan Y, Gotsman I, Pines M, Beinart R, Zeira M, Ohana M, et al. Induction of oral tolerance in splenocyte recipients toward pretransplant antigens ameliorates chronic graft versus host disease in a murine model. *Blood* 2000; 95(11):3613–9.

14. Nagler A, Pines M, Abadi U, Pappo O, Zeira M, Rabbani E, et al. Oral tolerization ameliorates liver disorders associated with chronic graft versus host disease in mice. *Hepatology* 2000; 31(3):641–8.

15. Ilan Y, Prakash R, Davidson A, Jona V, Droguett G, Horwitz MS, et al. Oral tolerization to adenoviral antigens permits long-term gene expression using recombinant adenoviral vectors. *J Clin Invest* 1997; 99(5):1098–106.

16. Morita H, Sugiura K, Inaba M, Jin T, Ishikawa J, Lian Z, et al. A strategy for organ allografts without using immunosuppressants or irradiation. *Proc Natl Acad Sci USA* 1998; 95(12):6947–52.

17. Opelz G, Margreiter R, Dohler B. Prolongation of long-term kidney graft survival by a simultaneous liver transplant: The liver does it, and the heart does it too. *Transplantation* 2002; 74(10):1390–4.

18. Starzl TE, Murase N, Demetris A, Trucco M, Fung J. The mystique of hepatic tolerogenicity. *Semin Liver Dis* 2000; 20(4):497–510.

19. Meyer D, Otto C, Rummel C, Gassel HJ, Timmermann W, Ulrichs K, et al. "Tolerogenic effect" of the liver for a small bowel allograft. *Transpl Int* 2000; 13(Suppl 1):S123–S126.

20. Sarnacki S, Revillon Y, Cerf-Bensussan N, Calise D, Goulet O, Brousse N. Long-term small-bowel graft survival induced by a spontaneously tolerated liver allograft in inbred rat strains. *Transplantation* 1992; 54(2):383–5.

21. Kamada N, Wight DG. Antigen-specific immunosuppression induced by liver transplantation in the rat. *Transplantation* 1984; 38(3):217–21.

22. Eason JD, Cohen AJ, Nair S, Alcantera T, Loss GE. Tolerance: Is it worth the risk? *Transplantation* 2005; 79(9):1157–9.

23. Adams AB, Williams MA, Jones TR, Shirasugi N, Durham MM, Kaech SM, et al. Heterologous immunity provides a potent barrier to transplantation tolerance. *J Clin Invest* 2003; 111(12):1887–95.

24. Lorenz EN. Deterministic nonperiodic flow. *J Atm Sci* 1963; 20:130–41.

25. Li TY, Yorke JA. Period three implies chaos. *Am Math Monthly* 1975; 82:985.

26. Racanelli V, Rehermann B. The liver as an immunological organ. *Hepatology* 2006; 43(2 Suppl 1):S54–S62.

27. Lau AH, Thomson AW. Dendritic cells and immune regulation in the liver. *Gut* 2003; 52(2):307–14.

28. Sanchez-Fueyo A, Strom TB. Immunological tolerance and liver transplantation. *J Hepatol* 2004; 41(5):698–705.

29. Pahlavan PS, Feldmann RE, Jr., Zavos C, Kountouras J. Prometheus' challenge: Molecular, cellular and systemic aspects of liver regeneration. *J Surg Res* 2006; 134(2): 238–51.

30. Wisse E, Gregoriadis G, Daems WT. Electron microscopic cytochemical localization of intravenously injected liposome-encapsulated horseradish peroxidase in rat liver cells. *Adv Exp Med Biol* 1976; 73(Pt A):237–45.

31. Wisse E. Ultrastructure and function of Kupffer cells and other sinusoidal cells in the liver. *Med Chir Dig* 1977; 6(7):409–18.

32. Wisse E, De Zanger RB, Charels K, Van Der SP, McCuskey RS. The liver sieve: Considerations concerning the structure and function of endothelial fenestrae, the sinusoidal wall and the space of Disse. *Hepatology* 1985; 5(4):683–92.

33. Onoe T, Ohdan H, Tokita D, Shishida M, Tanaka Y, Hara H, et al. Liver sinusoidal endothelial cells tolerize T cells across MHC barriers in mice. *J Immunol* 2005; 175(1):139–46.

34. Onoe T, Ohdan H, Tokita D, Hara H, Tanaka Y, Ishiyama K, et al. Liver sinusoidal endothelial cells have a capacity for inducing nonresponsiveness of T cells across major histocompatibility complex barriers. *Transpl Int* 2005; 18(2):206–14.

35. Bowen DG, Zen M, Holz L, Davis T, McCaughan GW, Bertolino P. The site of primary T cell activation is a determinant of the balance between intrahepatic tolerance and immunity. *J Clin Invest* 2004; 114(5):701–12.

36. Wick MJ, Leithauser F, Reimann J. The hepatic immune system. *Crit Rev Immunol* 2002; 22(1):47–103.

37. Dini L, Lentini A, Diez GD, Rocha M, Falasca L, Serafino L, et al. Phagocytosis of apoptotic bodies by liver endothelial cells. *J Cell Sci* 1995; 108(Pt 3):967–73.

38. Steffan AM, Gendrault JL, McCuskey RS, McCuskey PA, Kirn A. Phagocytosis, an unrecognized property of murine endothelial liver cells. *Hepatology* 1986; 6(5):830–6.

39. Limmer A, Ohl J, Kurts C, Ljunggren HG, Reiss Y, Groettrup M, et al. Efficient presentation of exogenous antigen by liver endothelial cells to CD8+ T cells results in antigen-specific T-cell tolerance. *Nat Med* 2000; 6(12):1348–54.

40. Knolle PA, Gerken G, Loser E, Dienes HP, Gantner F, Tiegs G, et al. Role of sinusoidal endothelial cells of the liver in concanavalin A-induced hepatic injury in mice. *Hepatology* 1996; 24(4):824–9.

41. Knolle P, Schlaak J, Uhrig A, Kempf P, Meyer zum Buschenfelde KH, Gerken G. Human Kupffer cells secrete IL-10 in response to lipopolysaccharide (LPS) challenge. *J Hepatol* 1995; 22(2):226–9.

42. Groux H, Bigler M, de Vries JE, Roncarolo MG. Interleukin-10 induces a long-term antigen-specific anergic state in human CD4+ T cells. *J Exp Med* 1996; 184(1):19–29.

43. Bertolino P, McCaughan GW, Bowen DG. Role of primary intrahepatic T-cell activation in the "liver tolerance effect." *Immunol Cell Biol* 2002; 80(1):84–92.

44. Crispe IN, Dao T, Klugewitz K, Mehal WZ, Metz DP. The liver as a site of T-cell apoptosis: Graveyard, or killing field? *Immunol Rev* 2000; 174:47–62.

45. Scherer MN, Graeb C, Tange S, Dyson C, Jauch KW, Geissler EK. Immunologic considerations for therapeutic strategies utilizing allogeneic hepatocytes: Hepatocyte-expressed membrane-bound major histocompatibility complex class I antigen sensitizes while soluble antigen suppresses the immune response in rats. *Hepatology* 2000; 32(5):999–1007.

46. Behrens D, Lange K, Fried A, Yoo-Ott KA, Richter K, Fandrich F, et al. Donor-derived soluble MHC antigens plus low-dose cyclosporine induce transplantation unresponsiveness independent of the thymus by down-regulating T cell-mediated alloresponses in a rat transplantation model. *Transplantation* 2001; 72(12): 1974–82.

47. Tang H, McLachlan A. Transcriptional regulation of hepatitis B virus by nuclear hormone receptors is a critical determinant of viral tropism. *Proc Natl Acad Sci USA* 2001; 98(4):1841–6.

48. Ishikawa T, Ganem D. The pre-S domain of the large viral envelope protein determines host range in avian hepatitis B viruses. *Proc Natl Acad Sci USA* 1995; 92(14):6259–63.

49. Yamaguchi Y, Tsumura H, Miwa M, Inaba K. Contrasting effects of TGF-beta 1 and TNF-alpha on the development of dendritic cells from progenitors in mouse bone marrow. *Stem Cells* 1997; 15(2):144–53.

50. Steinbrink K, Wolfl M, Jonuleit H, Knop J, Enk AH. Induction of tolerance by IL-10-treated dendritic cells. *J Immunol* 1997; 159(10):4772–80.

51. Thomson AW, Lu L, Murase N, Demetris AJ, Rao AS, Starzl TE. Microchimerism, dendritic cell progenitors and transplantation tolerance. *Stem Cells* 1995; 13(6):622–39.

52. Starzl TE, Demetris AJ, Rao AS, Thomson AW, Trucco M, Murase N. Migratory nonparenchymal cells after organ allotransplantation: With particular reference to chimerism and the liver. *Prog Liver Dis* 1994; 12:191–213.

53. Starzl TE, Demetris AJ, Trucco M, Murase N, Ricordi C, Ildstad S, et al. Cell migration and chimerism after whole-organ transplantation: The basis of graft acceptance. *Hepatology* 1993; 17(6):1127–52.

54. Exley MA, Koziel MJ. To be or not to be NKT: Natural killer T cells in the liver. *Hepatology* 2004; 40(5):1033–40.

55. de Creus A, Abe M, Lau AH, Hackstein H, Raimondi G, Thomson AW. Low TLR4 expression by liver dendritic cells correlates with reduced capacity to activate allogeneic T cells in response to endotoxin. *J Immunol* 2005; 174(4): 2037–45.

56. Limmer A, Knolle PA. Liver sinusoidal endothelial cells: A new type of organ-resident antigen-presenting cell. *Arch Immunol Ther Exp (Warsz)* 2001; 49(Suppl 1):S7–S11.

57. Xu H, Zhang X, Mannon RB, Kirk AD. Platelet-derived or soluble CD154 induces vascularized allograft rejection independent of cell-bound CD154. *J Clin Invest* 2006; 116(3):769–74.

58. Billingham RE, Brent L, Medawar PB. Activity acquired tolerance of foreign cells. *Nature* 1953; 172(4379):603–6.

59. Mazariegos GV, Ramos H, Shapiro R, Zeevi A, Fung JJ, Starzl TE. Weaning of immunosuppression in long-term recipients of living related renal transplants: A preliminary study. *Transpl Proc* 1995; 27(1):207–9.

60. Devlin J, Doherty D, Thomson L, Wong T, Donaldson P, Portmann B, et al. Defining the outcome of immunosuppression withdrawal after liver transplantation. *Hepatology* 1998; 27(4):926–33.

61. Girlanda R, Rela M, Williams R, O'Grady JG, Heaton ND. Long-term outcome of immunosuppression withdrawal after liver transplantation. *Transpl Proc* 2005; 37(4):1708–9.

62. Inomata Y, Hamamoto R, Yoshimoto K, Zeledon M. [Current status and perspective of pediatric liver transplantation in Japan.] *Nippon Rinsho* 2005; 63(11):1986–92.

63. Ueda M, Koshiba T, Li Y, Pirenne J, Inazawa Y, Egawa H, et al. Requirement of protocol biopsy before and after complete cessation of immunosuppression following living-donor liver transplantation. *Am J Transpl* 2005; 5(11):374.

64. Pons JA, Yelamos J, Ramirez P, Oliver-Bonet M, Sanchez A, Rodriguez-Gago M, et al. Endothelial cell chimerism does not influence allograft tolerance in liver transplant patients after withdrawal of immunosuppression. *Transplantation* 2003; 75(7):1045–7.

65. Calne R. WOFIE hypothesis: Some thoughts on an approach toward allograft tolerance. *Transpl Proc* 1996; 28(3):1152.

2

Novel Approaches to Immunosuppression in Liver Transplantation

Christian Toso, MD, Andrew L. Mason, MB, BS, and Norman M. Kneteman, MD, MSc, MSM

CONTENTS

Abstract

In recent years, a variety of immunosuppressive (IS) agents has emerged. The best application and combination of these new agents along with traditional immunosuppressive agents present challenges

From: *Clinical Gastroenterology: Liver Transplantation: Challenging Controversies and Topics*
Edited by: G. T. Everson and J. F. Trotter, DOI: 10.1007/978-1-60327-028-1_2,
© Humana Press, Totowa, NJ

and opportunities to transplant physicians. Two anti-IL2 receptor monoclonal antibodies are currently available for clinical use: daclizumab (Zenapax, Roche) and basiliximab (Simulect, Novartis). Both bind to the alpha subunit of the IL-2 receptor (CD-25), which is expressed on activated, but not resting, lymphocytes. These drugs are the most commonly used induction agents in the United States. Campath-1H (C-1H) or alemtuzumab (Ilex Pharmaceuticals) has been used in a limited fashion in liver transplantation recipients, with mixed results. The role of sirolimus in liver transplantation remains controversial. However, this agent may offer specific advantages in patients with hepatocellular carcinoma or renal dysfunction. Because hepatitis C is the most common indication for liver transplantation, the application of immunosuppression in these patients is important. However, the best regimen for these patients remains controversial. The role of new immunosuppressive drugs including FTY720, FK778, and LEA29Y offers the promise for better immunosuppression for future liver transplantation recipients.

Key Words: Immunosuppression; Interleukin receptor antagonist; Campath; Sirolimus; Hepatitis C; Hepatocellular carcinoma

INTRODUCTION

Two decades ago, a narrow selection of immunosuppressive options was available for clinical application. As a result, liver graft recipients received a limited variation of cyclosporine-based regimens. Within recent years, a variety of selective and usually more potent agents has become available for clinicians, facilitating the development of a myriad of different drug combinations. The wealth of choice for immunosuppression (IS) regimens has coincided with new challenges for the transplant community, resulting in the tailoring of regimens to suit different organs, specific diseases, and even individual recipients. We now have the opportunity to achieve effective IS for specific transplant-related diseases, with the view to minimizing side effects for individuals at risk.

With the exception of hepatitis C virus (HCV) infection, data are lacking to suggest that single, treated rejection episodes adversely impact the long-term outcome after liver transplantation (1). Accordingly, protocols directed toward achieving single-digit rates of rejection following liver transplantation are perhaps less desirable than in other arenas of transplantation where acute rejection is associated with demonstrable deterioration in long-term graft function (2). Medical management of liver transplant recipients has evolved, accordingly, to address morbidity and mortality related to the adverse effects of IS rather than the efficacy of specific IS regimens. The change in focus has occurred as a result of the increased debility of patients waiting longer for liver transplantation and the expanded use of living related donors and the cadaveric donor pool. Apart from the recognized increase in infectious and neoplastic disease, the major side effects of IS predominantly include nephrotoxicity, neurotoxicity, osteoporosis, delayed wound healing, diabetes, dyslipidemia, hypertension, and cardiovascular and cerebrovascular disease. The majority of these side effects are related to calcineurin inhibitor and corticosteroid use; regimens that limit the treatment with these agents, while focusing on specific needs for individual patients, provide a more directional approach to IS in liver transplant recipients.

This chapter provides an update on newly available and clinically relevant but established IS agents as well as emergent therapies with promise for future impact. The advantages and disadvantages of selected potential applications are also discussed with a view to establishing IS regimens tailored for specific patient populations with renal, viral, immune-related, and neoplastic disease.

ANTI-IL-2 RECEPTOR (ANTI-CD25) MONOCLONAL ANTIBODIES

Two anti-IL-2 receptor monoclonal antibodies are currently available for clinical use: daclizumab (Zenapax, Roche) and basiliximab (Simulect, Novartis). Both bind to the alpha subunit of the IL-2 receptor (CD-25), which is expressed on activated, but not resting, lymphocytes. As a result, the subunit of the receptor is internalized and IL-2 can only bind with very low affinity.

These antibodies induce virtually no side effects, in contrast to alternative induction compounds such as OKT3 or anti-thymocyte globulins (3–5). According to the 2003 report of the Scientific Registry of Transplant Recipients (www.ustransplant.org), anti-IL-2 receptor antibodies are the induction drugs most commonly used in the United States, with 12.7% of all liver recipients receiving one of them.

Daclizumab

Daclizumab is a genetically engineered mouse antibody that has been modified to have 90% human component. As a result, the incidence of acute hypersensitivity reactions is negligible. The risk of anti-idiotypic antibodies is minimal, allowing repeated injections without risk of decreased efficiency (6). This approach has been found to be effective in islet transplantation, for example, where courses of daclizumab induction are required for repeated islet infusion without increased risk of rejection following the most recent transplantation (7).

In vitro and *in vivo* data suggest that serum levels of 5 to 10 ng/mL are necessary to saturate the alpha subunit. Injection at 1 mg/kg is efficient for approximately 90 days in adults, with an estimated elimination half-life of 20 days (manufacturer's data). In liver transplant recipients, however, the elimination can be accelerated with drainage of antibody in protein-rich ascitic fluid (6). The drug was originally designed to be used every second week for five administrations but, in recent clinical application in liver transplantation, it is most often used with two injections only, with the second 4 to 14 days after transplantation (8–10).

Daclizumab was approved in 1997 by the FDA to be used in conjunction with a standard course of immunosuppressive therapy in kidney recipients. It was the first monoclonal antibody to achieve a treatment label for prevention of rejection, as OKT3 was originally approved for the treatment of acute rejection rather than prophylaxis. Studies in liver transplant recipients showed that daclizumab prophylaxis reduced the rate of acute cellular rejection. A nonrandomized study at the University of Pennsylvania using daclizumab induction reported less acute rejection episodes compared to no induction in patients maintained on calcineurin inhibitors (CNI)/mycophenolate mofetil (MMF)/steroids, (11, 12). These findings were confirmed by a second study using a similar protocol, but with a single dose of daclizumab at 2 mg/kg (13). In comparison to a historical control group receiving OKT3 prophylaxis, patients treated with daclizumab demonstrated similar rates of acute rejection (4).

More recently, anti-IL-2 receptor monoclonal antibody therapy has been used to study early tapering of other IS therapy. One pilot study reported that a completely CNI-free daclizumab/MMF/steroid regimen was associated with a high rate of acute cellular rejection (7/7 recipients) (14), suggesting that anti-IL-2 antibody therapy was insufficient to attempt CNI-free protocols for the induction and maintenance of liver transplantation in the absence of other modifications. However, daclizumab induction has been used to introduce CNI therapy at lower doses rather than eliminate CNI in liver transplant recipients. For example, in a multicenter trial, Yoshida and colleagues compared daclizumab with a 4- to 6-day delay in starting low-dose tacrolimus to standard-dose tacrolimus/MMF ($n = 72$ vs. 76) with tapering steroids in both groups; patients with significant renal dysfunction prior to transplant were excluded. While acute rejection rates and graft and patient survivals were similar in both groups, the cohort with daclizumab induction had significantly higher glomerular filtration rates within the first week and at both one and six months' posttransplant (10). Even though the statistical significance of the differences was lost with longer follow-up in this study, early renal function appears as a key predictive factor of longer-term renal outcome (15). The benefit of using daclizumab induction with delayed introduction of low-dose CNI seems a logical choice for patients with impaired renal function at the time of transplantation. Daclizumab induction has also been utilized successfully in steroid avoidance strategies. For example, in one multicenter, randomized trial comparing daclizumab/tacrolimus to corticosteroids/tacrolimus (n = 351 vs. 347), the mean maintenance tacrolimus trough levels were comparable in both study arms (10.6 vs. 10.9 ng/mL) and the patient and graft survival and the incidence of acute rejection were also similar (9). However, the steroid/tacrolimus group experienced an increased frequency of steroid-resistant episodes and had significantly higher rates of diabetes mellitus (15.3% vs. 5.7%) and cytomegalovirus infection (11.5% vs. 5.1%) as compared to the daclizumab/tacrolimus patients. As observed in comparable studies (8), the steroid-free patients experienced improved bone mineral density and triglyceride levels and none developed hypercholesterolemia, while 16% of steroid/tacrolimus patients did.

The impact of anti-CD25 induction therapy on the incidence and severity of HCV recurrence post liver transplant continues to be controversial. A nonrandomized study including steroid treatment in both arms reported earlier onset of hepatitis and jaundice and worse histological score in the daclizumab-treated group as compared to historical controls (16). However, a preliminary report of a randomized study comparing daclizumab and corticosteroid therapy contradicted these results, as both treatment arms maintained on tacrolimus/MMF had similar outcomes (17). While further studies are required, it seems reasonable to speculate that daclizumab does not provide an increased risk for HCV recurrence when substituted for another agent but may do so as an additional agent providing an increased burden of IS.

The high upfront costs of the anti-CD25 antibodies may limit their wider use. On balance, however, patients experience fewer complications than with full-dose CNI or steroid-containing IS protocols. As such, it is likely that the overall cost of transplantation is comparable when anti-CD25 antibodies are used to limit the side effects of full-dose CNI and corticosteroid therapy. The administration of only two doses of daclizumab, instead of the recommended five doses, provides an additional option to reduce costs further. Using this strategy in kidney recipients, $715 can be saved per patient without increasing the risk of acute cellular rejection (18).

Basiliximab

Basiliximab is a chimeric antibody including variable regions of a murine anti-CD25 monoclonal antibody and constant regions of human immunoglobulin G1 heavy and K light chains. While its structure theoretically presents a higher risk of anti-idiotypic antibody development than daclizumab, anti-basiliximab antibodies have not yet been detected in clinical use (19).

Basiliximab has a half-life of nine days. At the recommended dose of 20 mg on the day of transplantation and four days later, receptor-saturating concentrations were maintained for approximately 38 days (20). The rate of antibody loss is increased during bleeding episodes; the first dose should not be administrated until the risk of operative blood loss has been controlled (21). Also, up to 20% of clearance may occur through paracentesis of ascites; a supplemental dose should be considered for patients with more than 10 L of postoperative ascitic fluid drainage (20).

The FDA approved basiliximab in 1998 for the prophylaxis of solid organ graft rejection. In liver transplant recipients, basiliximab appears equivalent to daclizumab induction in reducing rates of acute liver rejection. In a randomized, multicenter trial, two-dose basiliximab was compared to placebo ($n = 188$ vs. 193), with cyclosporine and steroids in both groups (3). The rate of rejection episodes was significantly reduced in the basiliximab group at 6 months after transplantation and the trend remained at 12 months, although no longer reaching significance. Of note, the basiliximab arm experienced a significant reduction in biopsy-confirmed rejection, HCV recurrence, graft loss, or death at 6 and 12 months.

Preliminary results in the pediatric transplant population suggest that basiliximab can be used as rescue therapy for acute rejection (22). While basiliximab has also shown utility for acute rejection in an adult case report (23), more rigorous studies will be required to determine the potential impact. Basiliximab has been successfully employed in renal transplant recipients to provide a "CNI holiday" and also to study the potential for minimizing the side effects of CNI and steroids in liver transplantation. In a corticosteroid-free combination with low-dose tacrolimus and MMF, the rate of acute cellular rejection, new-onset diabetes, CMV antigenemia, and hypercholesterolemia were all reduced with basiliximab versus corticosteroid therapy (24), paralleling outcomes with daclizumab outlined above.

As with daclizumab, the benefits of basiliximab have not yet been established in HCV-positive recipients. Neuhaus and colleagues reported similar rates of acute rejection with and without basiliximab induction in a placebo-controlled study (3) that were comparable to historical studies (5). However, others have found similar but less aggressive hepatitis C histological recurrence when steroids were avoided in a double-blind study comparing basiliximab/corticosteroids versus basiliximab/placebo with cyclosporine and azathioprine in both groups (25).

CAMPATH-1H

Campath-1H (C-1H), or alemtuzumab (Ilex Pharmaceuticals), is a humanized, recombinant anti-CD52 monoclonal antibody. CD52 is found on thymocytes, lymphocytes, NK cells, monocytes, and macrophages. C-1H induces a sharp depletion of these cells for approximately one month, with a very slow recovery in lymphocyte populations that may take over a year to normalize (26). In clinical studies, idiotypic antibodies are seldom detected, allowing repeated courses of treatment (27). C-1H has been evaluated in lymphoid malignancies, rheumatoid arthritis, and multiple sclerosis.

In renal transplantation, the combination of C-1H with cyclosporine monotherapy has similar rejection and survival rates to historical controls treated with CNI/azathioprine/corticosteroid therapy. The rejection episodes appeared later than that observed in the historical control groups, probably reflecting the clearance of C-1H with time (28). Of note, the combination of C-1H with rapamycin maintenance monotherapy was associated with high rates of rejection, with one fourth of the patients requiring conversion to a conventional triple therapy for graft salvage (29).

In liver transplant recipients, the combination of Campath and tacrolimus has been evaluated using a historical control group treated with a tacrolimus and corticosteroid regimen ($n = 40$ vs. 50). C-1H was administrated at 0.3 mg/kg just before and after the transplant procedure, and on day 3 and day 7. Rejection, patient survival, and graft survival rates were similar, but patients in the C-1H group received fewer maintenance steroids and lower doses of tacrolimus, resulting in significantly lower creatinine levels (30). In hepatitis C–positive recipients, a single 30-mg dose of C-1H was associated with a high risk of HCV recurrence after transplantation (26). At present, there are insufficient data concerning the use of Campath in liver graft recipients to guide clinical practice. C-1H in combination with low-dose CNI has the potential to maintain satisfactory control of the alloimmune response and is currently being evaluated by the Immune Tolerance Network in a complete IS withdrawal protocol. In liver transplant recipients with HCV infection, lymphocyte-depleting antibodies are not recommended for the treatment of rejection, and their role in prophylaxis continues to be debated (31).

The major side effects of Campath-1H are related to its hematological toxicity, including autoimmune idiopathic thrombocytopenic purpura, pancytopenia, marrow hypoplasia, and autoimmune hemolytic anemia. These risks are especially evident with single doses of C-1H greater than 30 mg and cumulative doses greater than 90 mg per week (www.fda.org).

The induction of prolonged suppression of lymphocyte counts mandates further careful long-term follow-up given the potential for an increase in malignancy with such impact (32).

RAPAMYCIN

Rapamycin (sirolimus, Rapamune, Wyeth) is a macrolide antibiotic, structurally related to tacrolimus. The named was derived from Rapa Nui, a region of Easter Island, where rapamycin was first isolated from soil samples returned by the Canadian geological expedition. It was originally reported as an fungicidal antibiotic (33).

Sirolimus acts by forming an active complex with a cytosolic immunophyllin—the FK binding protein 12—but unlike the CNI, this has little effect on inhibiting the signal 1 MHC/T cell receptor pathway that leads to nuclear factor of activated T cell (NFAT) initiation. Rather, the sirolimus/FKBP12 complex negatively regulates kinases referred to as mammalian targets-of-rapamycin (m-TOR) that leads to blockade of the B7-1/B7-2 to CD28 costimulatory signal 2 pathway interfering with NF-KB–induced secretion of IL-2 and other cytokines (34); and abrogation of the signal 3 signal transduction pathway from cytokine/growth factor receptors to the nucleus to initiate cell cycling and proliferation (35).

The U.S. Food and Drug Administration approved sirolimus in 1999 for its use in kidney recipients in combination with cyclosporine and corticosteroids. Sirolimus has also found a niche in the management of liver transplant recipients with hepatocellular carcinoma, renal insufficiency, and other CNI-related toxicity. However, the role of sirolimus in liver transplantation remains controversial. In multicenter phase II/III trials, the combination of sirolimus with CNI and steroids was reportedly as good as or better than classical CNI and steroids regimens in preventing rejection (36, 37). In nonrandomized, single-center trials, sirolimus combinations with reduced tacrolimus dosing reported frequency of acute cellular rejection at least equal to historical control groups (38–41).

Sirolimus and Side Effects in Liver Recipients

In two multicenter phase II/III trials (36, 37), sirolimus was associated with a trend to increased rates of hepatic artery thrombosis (HAT) within the first three weeks of transplant. Although the Data Safety Monitoring Boards reported that technical and donor factors were partly responsible for the HAT, the sponsor cancelled both trials. The second of these studies also demonstrated an increased risk of graft loss and death in the sirolimus/tacrolimus combination group, which was likely due, in part, to high serum levels achieved for both potent IS agents. As a result, the FDA subsequently mandated a "Black Box" warning around the use of rapamycin stipulating that it does not recommend the use of rapamycin in liver transplant recipients, especially soon after transplantation.

In contrast, no increased thrombotic events were reported in kidney transplantation trials with sirolimus, nor in uncontrolled but large liver transplant case series. The University of Colorado reported similar rates of HAT in 170 patients treated from date of transplant with rapamycin, compared to historical control patients (39). The Dalhousie University series had only one case of thrombosis out of 56 liver recipients (40). In our series of 63 consecutive patients with hepatocellular carcinoma treated with sirolimus from the time of transplantation, three patients presented with arterial stenosis, but none developed HAT (41). While these single-center reports provide a degree of reassurance with rapamycin usage in liver transplantation, the trend of increased rates of HAT in two consecutive randomized clinical trials mandates caution with sirolimus therapy in the first few weeks posttransplant.

Sirolimus slows wound healing, as predicted by the mechanism of action. Although the University of Colorado series did not report an increase in wound complications, we and others have experienced high rates of wound healing complications and incisional hernias, approaching 30% of patients now in long-term follow-up (36, 40, 41). This has been especially troublesome in patients treated with both sirolimus and steroids, where a prolonged delay in wound healing has been observed.

Patients treated with sirolimus have experienced several other side effects including anemia and leukopenia, diabetes and dyslipidemia, lower extremity edema, dermatitis, joint pain, and pleural effusion (41, 42). Dyslipidemia appears less troublesome when sirolimus is combined with tacrolimus rather than cyclosporine (43). Although self-limiting with dose reduction, mouth ulcers appear in approximately 25% of patients irrespective of corticosteroid use (42). They are painful and provide a significant cause of patient concern, especially in islet transplantation, where up to 90% of patients experience this problem (44).

On the whole, sirolimus appears to be very efficient in preventing rejection, with comparable efficacy to calcineurin inhibitors. Sirolimus allows the use of substantially reduced doses of CNI and steroids and, in some cases, their complete elimination (40, 41). Single-center studies suggest HAT problems may not be as common as initially thought, but the potential for such a devastating complication clearly requires careful observation. There are clinical conditions where sirolimus appears intuitively the best choice for patient care; our own approach to rapamycin therapy soon after transplantation includes the routine use of low-dose anticoagulation and documented, informed patient consent. Delayed wound healing is a clear concern that may require direct action such as delayed introduction of rapamycin or the use of permanent sutures.

Sirolimus for Liver Recipients with Hepatocellular Carcinoma (HCC)

United Network for Organ Sharing (UNOS) and additional registry data show an increased incidence of cancer after transplantation, likely due to the impact of immunosuppression on tumor surveillance and viral replication. Posttransplant lymphoproliferative disorders (PTLD) and skin cancers are the most frequently reported, but the risk of developing cancer is modulated by the choice of IS (45). While CNI and antibody preparations have been associated with an increased risk, m-TOR inhibitors appear associated with a reduced incidence of posttransplant malignancy (45–47). m-TOR inhibitors alone or combined with calcineurin inhibitors have a significantly decreased incidence of skin or solid cancers compared to other calcineurin inhibitor-based regimens (45).

Sirolimus is the most studied m-TOR inhibitor in this regard; its antitumor activity was reported in the mid-1980s (48). More recent reports have shown that sirolimus inhibits angiogenesis by interfering with VEGF-mediated pathways in endothelial cells, limiting the growth of tumors (49). It can also impact established tumor vessels by inducing extensive microthrombi, which have been found in tumor vasculature, but not in the surrounding vessels. The microthrombi are associated with an increased rapamycin-mediated tissue factor (TF) secretion by endothelial cells (50).

While sirolimus induces fewer de novo cancers than other immunosuppression drugs, it remains to be determined whether it can reduce the risk of posttransplant recurrence in patients with HCC. At the present time, most groups use the Milan criteria to restrict transplantation to patients with limited HCC, with one nodule up to 5 cm or three or fewer nodules less than 3 cm each (51). Several studies have confirmed that patients with HCC can achieve outstanding survival results after liver transplant using the Milan criteria (47). However, we hypothesized that the criteria may be overly restrictive by prohibiting access to transplant for a substantial number of patients with more advanced tumors who could possibly achieve comparable oncological and transplant outcomes. We therefore addressed the specific objectives to determine whether sirolimus could improve results in patients with HCC and permit an expansion beyond the Milan criteria.

In 1996, we began a pilot trial of consecutive HCC patients with a single tumor up to 7.5 cm in diameter or multiple tumors up to 5 cm in diameter, without restricting the number of tumors. Exclusion criteria included extrahepatic disease or major vascular invasion on imaging; candidates with tumors over 5 cm in diameter required preoperative biopsy to rule out high tumor grade, which, in combination with tumor size >5 cm, was considered unacceptable for transplant. At the time of transplantation, patients were put on a combination of sirolimus/low-dose calcineurin inhibitor. The first 21 patients received steroids for the first three months; the subsequent 42 patients were completely free of steroids, receiving a single dose of anti-IL-2 receptor antibodies for induction. After 46 months' mean follow-up, 6 patients out of 32 (18.8%) beyond Milan criteria experienced a recurrence, and 1 of 31 (3.2%) patients within the Milan criteria. After recurrence, mean survival was 25 ± 29 (SD) months, with a single patient experiencing recurrence at four years (who survived nine years after transplantation), without additional treatment apart from maintenance rapamycin at 10–12 ug/L. Actuarial patient survival at one and four years posttransplant in this sequential cohort pilot study was 86% and 84% in the Milan group and 79% and 76% in the extended criteria group. One- and four-year tumor-free survival rates were also similar in the two groups (log-rank test, $p = 0.15$; Fig. 1), with 86% and 77% of the Milan criteria patients compared to 70% and 62% of patients with extended criteria both alive and free of tumor.

Assessing the impact of sirolimus on tumor biology in a nonrandomized pilot series is challenging, but a few findings are pertinent to the standard of care for liver transplant patients with HCC. Sirolimus may offer an advantage to patients within the Milan criteria, as only 3% of our patients developed recurrence after 46 months mean follow-up

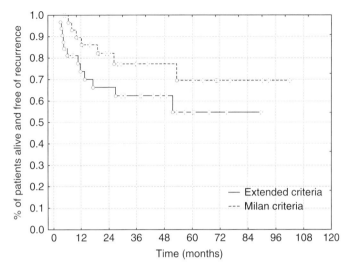

Fig. 1. Recurrence-free survival after liver transplantation in patients with hepatocellular carcinoma, with Milan criteria (31 patients) or with extended criteria (32 patients). All received a sirolimus-based immunosuppressive protocol with low-dose CNI tapered to discontinuation. Survival was similar in both groups (log-rank test, $p = 0.15$) and meets current outcome standards for candidacy for liver transplantation.

compared to recurrence rates of 11% reported with IS protocols using other drugs (51, 52). Also, while there was a trend toward worse outcome when the Milan criteria were extended, no statistical difference was found, albeit with a limited sample size. We can provide a degree of cautious optimism in contrast to previous studies showing a sharp decrease in patient tumor-free survival when Milan criteria were extended (51, 52). Further controlled trials will be required to establish whether there is clinical benefit from expanding the candidacy criteria for liver transplantation for patients with HCC with sirolimus maintenance therapy. Studies such as these will also allow us to assess whether sirolimus therapy provides additional benefit for patients with recurrent HCC as patients experienced 25 ($\pm$29) months mean survival following recurrence of HCC in our study.

There is a cautious optimism that sirolimus can provide additional benefit for liver transplant recipients with HCC. Our results to date have shown acceptable rates of one- and four-year patient survival with modest expansion of the Milan criteria. Clear evaluation of the impact of rapamycin in combination with steroid avoidance and CNI minimization in such patients awaits definitive randomized comparison.

Sirolimus for Liver Recipients with Renal Dysfunction

In kidney transplantation, the introduction of sirolimus maintenance treatment has provided the leeway to remove CNI therapy, which has resulted in improvement in renal function despite a modest increase in the rate of rejection (53). After liver transplantation, CNI replacement by sirolimus can also improve renal function in recipients with preexisting renal dysfunction (54, 55), where up to 71% of patients can improve glomerular filtration rate a year after substituting the CNI with rapamycin (55).

Even though sirolimus has a role in the management of liver recipients with renal dysfunction, a word of caution is required. Recently rapamycin has been linked with increased proteinuria or new-onset proteinuria after kidney and other organ transplantation (56, 57). Ongoing surveillance for proteinuria in rapamycin-treated transplant patients and evaluation of long-term impact on renal function will be required to better understand this potential challenge.

SDZ-RAD

SDZ-RAD, or everolimus (Certican, Novartis), is a close analogue of sirolimus with limited available data in liver transplantation to discuss this compound in detail. While it is likely to have similar impact, indications, and side effects as its close relative, sirolimus, it will be interesting to find out whether this agent is associated with HAT, limiting its use in liver transplant recipients. Everolimus has already been evaluated in renal transplantation with reduced doses of CNI to determine whether equivalent IS potency can be achieved with diminished overall side effects (58, 59). Everolimus is not yet labeled for use in North America nor in most countries.

COMPOUNDS IN DEVELOPMENT: FTY720, FK778, AND LEA29Y

FTY720 is a high-affinity agonist of the sphingosine-1-phosphate receptor-1. Once the ligand is bound to the receptor, the complex is internalized, with a net result of long-lasting inhibition of migration of the lymphocyte to lymphoid tissue. As a consequence, lymphocytes are unable to reach peripheral inflammatory tissues and graft sites once activated. Lymphopenia occurs without causing generalized suppression of cell function (60), which is reversed within three days after discontinuation of treatment (61).

FTY720's mechanism of action suggests the potential for synergistic impact when used with drugs such as cyclosporine, tacrolimus, sirolimus, or RAD. In combination with cyclosporine and steroids, FTY720 is associated with reduced frequency of acute rejection episodes in a dose-dependent fashion in kidney recipients (62). In animal models of liver transplantation, FTY720 can effectively prevent rejection (63) and reduce hepatic warm ischemia reperfusion injuries (64). Significant toxicity, including 15–20% bradycardia, has been reported in studies, however, limiting the use and development of this novel compound.

FK778 is a synthetic malononitrilamide, derived from the active metabolite of leflunomide. It has a shorter half-life than leflunomide (6–45 hours vs. 15–18 days) and inhibits both T cells and B cells by blocking de novo pyrimidine synthesis (65). Independent of the IS activity, FK778 appears able to block replication of several viruses including herpes family viruses, cytomegalovirus, and polyoma virus (65).

In a multicenter, randomized, double-blind trial, FK778/tacrolimus/steroids reduced the rate of acute rejection episodes when compared to placebo/tacrolimus/steroids in kidney recipients (66). In a rat liver allotransplantation model, FK778 alone or combined with tacrolimus prevented acute rejection and was effective in treating and rescuing ongoing acute rejections (67). While a phase II trial in liver transplantation in Europe and North America has been completed, no data have been presented or published to date.

LEA29Y, or belatacept, is a modified CTLA4-Ig, differing by two amino acids (L104E and A29Y). This compound blocks the signal 2 pathway of T cell activation by binding the B7-1/B7-2 or CD80/CD86 surface costimulatory ligands of antigen-presenting cells. It has a slow dissociation rate and a 10-fold increased *in vitro* potency compared to CTLA4-Ig. CTLA4-Ig has been shown to abrogate the immune response in various settings, including cell and solid organ transplantations and rheumatoid arthritis (68). LEA29Y therapy is associated with improved kidney graft outcomes in nonhuman primates when combined with MMF/steroids or basiliximab (69). In one study, LEA29Y used for de novo IS in kidney recipients has reportedly comparable rejection rates with cyclosporine used in combination with MMF and steroids (70).

According to animal experiments, costimulatory blockade tools can be successfully applied in liver transplantation, with outcomes similar to CNI (71). Such a strategy could potentially be applied to human liver transplantation, especially considering the association between CTLA4 gene polymorphisms and transplant outcome (72).

This molecule is among the most interesting new compounds with potential clinical applicability. A phase 2 trial in liver transplant is currently ongoing.

IMMUNOSUPPRESSION OF HCV-POSITIVE RECIPIENTS

HCV is the most common indication for liver transplantation in North America, affecting 40–50% of patients in most centers (73). Recurrence of HCV infection posttransplantation is universal and has become increasingly problematic over the last five years (74, 75). The increased shortage of organs and longer duration of waiting for liver transplantation have directly impacted the inferior outcomes that transplant recipients with HCV infection now experience. Factors directly associated with more severe HCV recurrence and with diminished graft and patient survival include increasingly deconditioned patients with renal insufficiency, the use of expanded donor range with more hepatic steatosis, longer cold ischemia, and grafts from older donors (31, 74, 75).

For HCV-positive recipients, it has also become clear that perturbations in IS result in more progressive liver disease. Therefore, IS should be targeted to achieve a balance to diminish the emergence of rampant HCV recurrence and replication as well as to avoid rejection episodes mandating marked fluctuation of IS therapy. It was been well established that bolus corticosteroid therapy and depleting antibodies, such as OKT3, for the treatment of rejection are associated with an adverse impact on long-term outcome (76–78). Indeed, HCV-positive recipients who experience a rejection have a threefold increased risk of death, a morbidity that is further increased with multiple steroid boluses (79) or when antibodies are required for antirejection treatment (80).

Although it remains subject to debate, corticosteroid maintenance therapy has an adverse impact on HCV recurrence rates (81–83). Two randomized studies have reported higher rates of aggressive HCV recurrence in the steroid-containing arms of protocols with anti-CD25 antibodies or tacrolimus (25, 84). Of interest, patients with corticosteroid induction after liver transplant have worse outcome with steroid withdrawal (85), underscoring the importance of IS stability as key factor in the HCV-infected patient posttransplant. While some proponents advocate the use of low-dose corticosteroids to ameliorate side effects of other IS agents, the aggregate data suggest that cumulative exposure to corticosteroids is associated with increased HCV viremia, worse histological recurrence, and higher mortality (31).

Mycophenolate mofetil (MMF) is a potent IS agent with anti-HCV activity; however, the role of MMF therapy on HCV recurrence in transplant recipients is controversial. In a study from Berlin, switching patients from azathioprine to MMF failed to show any reduction in HCV titers (86), and others have suggested that patients only benefit from high-dose MMF, as those maintained on lower doses actually faired worse than controls (87). However, a major study analyzing 11,670 patients from the Scientific Registry of Transplant Recipients clearly came out in favor of MMF use in patients with and without HCV. Patients administered MMF in conjunction with tacrolimus and steroids achieved better graft and patient survival when compared to MMF-free patients (88). However, a small randomized study ($n = 50$ vs. 56) was unable to reach the same conclusion, where no demonstrable improvement was shown in the rates of recurrence, graft, or patient survivals in subjects treated with MMF, tacrolimus, and steroids compared to tacrolimus and steroids alone (89). Others have championed older compounds, like azathioprine and corticosteroids, in a review of their retrospective analyses of 15-year outcomes (90). Once again, it is difficult to compare these studies, as many factors impact outcomes, including the impact of organ shortage, donor age, relative potency of IS combinations, the potential antiviral effects of MMF and other compounds, as well as other unknown factors that may have affected survival over a 15-year period. For our practice, we use steroid-free regimens with MMF for patients with HCV infection to minimize side effects and avoid the IS fluctuations of treating rejection.

Not surprisingly, the choice of calcineurin inhibitor for HCV-infected transplant recipients is a contentious issue as well. The worsening clinical outcomes of transplant patients with HCV infection and decreased survival reported in recent years by Berenguer and others (74) have led to speculation that the transition from cyclosporine-based to predominantly tacrolimus-based immunosuppression may be at least in part responsible. Cyclosporine exerts its immunosuppressive effect by binding cyclophilins, which inhibit signal 1 pathway by blocking NFAT, IL-2 secretion, and T cell activation. However, cyclophilins are peptidyl-prolyl isomerases required for a variety of other cellular processes involved in protein folding, trafficking, and secretion as well as mitochondrial function and transcriptional regulation, to name a few. Cyclosporine therefore has several well-documented antiviral effects against vaccinia, herpes simplex, and HIV by blocking the cellular activity of cyclophilins (91). For example, cyclosporine inhibits viral production by blocking the incorporation of cyclophilin into HIV particles and is required for HIV Gag protein assembly.

The ability of cyclosporine and nonimmunosuppressive analogues to inhibit HCV replication *in vitro* is well established (91, 92). An elegant series of experiments by Watashi and Nakagawa have outlined one mechanism of HCV inhibition by cyclosporine binding to cyclophilin B (93, 94). Cyclophilin B is a functional regulator of the HCV RNA polymerase required for HCV replication *in vivo* and in replicon cells *in vitro*. This cyclophilin binds the HCV NS5B protein to activate the RNA binding activity, which cyclosporine directly inhibits (93, 94).

The clinical impact of cyclosporine for patients with HCV infection can only be inferred from clinical observation, as the antiviral and immunosuppressive effects are difficult to separate in transplant patients. In combination with interferon-α, cyclosporine has been reported to provide additional benefit in nontransplant HCV-infected patients (95, 96) as well as in bone marrow transplant patients (97). A recent study of recipients receiving combination antiviral therapy with interferon-α and ribavirin reported a significant twofold increase (46% vs. 27%) in viral clearance in patients treated with cyclosporine-based IS as compared to those maintained with tacrolimus (98). This is potentially a very important finding if these data can be reproduced, as virological clearance in transplant recipients receiving cyclosporine is equilibrating toward what may be observed in patients prior to transplantation.

In liver transplant studies of patients with HCV infection, however, evidence supportive of the suggestion that cyclosporine provides clinically relevant patient and graft survival benefit as compared to tacrolimus has been difficult to find (99). Only one small randomized trial has been performed as a head-to-head comparison of cyclosporine and tacrolimus in patients with HCV infection, but, not surprisingly, similar HCV recurrence and survival rates were observed in this small study (100). In a larger study not specifically conducted to assess HCV infection, the subgroup of patients with HCV recurrence experienced inferior patient survival and greater graft loss with tacrolimus as compared to cyclosporine (15% vs. 6%) (101). However, studies that are not specifically directed toward comparing outcomes in patients with HCV infection are difficult to interpret.

Sirolimus has also demonstrated a potential for benefit for patients with HCV infection, albeit in a very preliminary recent report. Two liver recipients who were put on this drug because of renal dysfunction cleared serum HCV RNA without antiviral treatment (102). Larger studies with longer follow-up that are directly addressed to the study of HCV infection will be required for clarification of whether either cyclosporine or sirolimus provides superior outcomes compared to tacrolimus. It is interesting to note that this phenomenon is not just related to patients with recurrent HCV infection following transplantation. In a large retrospective study from the University of Birmingham, recurrent primary biliary cirrhosis was observed to occur significantly earlier and more aggressively in patients taking tacrolimus as compared to cyclosporine as their primary immunosuppression (103). These data have not been replicated, but the implication of an infectious etiology of primary biliary cirrhosis that may be responsive to a cyclophilin inhibitor is tantalizing. We eagerly anticipate the clinical development of nonimmunosuppressive cyclosporine analogues with antiviral activity for HCV infection.

While it appears clear that injudicious use of potent immunosuppressive therapies can significantly worsen the posttransplant course of recurrent HCV disease, it remains to be demonstrated that variations on existing immunosuppressive protocols hold the key to control of HCV recurrence following liver transplantation. As recently described (98), the tailoring of cyclosporine with antiviral therapy appears intuitive, but further studies will be required to clearly demonstrate their utility. Side effects of antiviral therapy provide one of the major obstacles for the management of HCV infection in liver transplant patients. Fortunately, the development of new systems for study of HCV infection, including the replicon viral constructs (104), cell culture (105, 106), and small animal models (107), have helped in the progress to clinical evaluation of a series of promising new anti-HCV therapeutics. This new generation holds promise for substantial improvements in HCV control compared to the rather limited performance of pegylated interferon-α and ribavirin in the posttransplant patient with HCV recurrence. Of note, newer antiviral regimens suggest that a cure is not an unrealistic goal despite the impact of ongoing immunosuppression.

PROSPECTUS

With the use of a range of immunosuppressive agents currently available, we seldom experience graft loss as a result of rejection in compliant individuals. At the University of Alberta, only 3 liver grafts out of 803 transplants (0.4%) were lost because of acute rejection between 1991 and 2005. Chronic rejection has also become a relatively minor challenge in liver transplant programs: Only 8 of 803 liver transplants (1%) in our own program have been lost to chronic rejection over the last 15 years. However, three major challenges remain with regard to immunosuppression. The first is balancing effective antirejection therapy with the risk of infection and sepsis after liver transplant, especially in the critically ill before and after transplantation, or those suffering a major technical complication postoperatively. A further obstacle is the emerging impact of recurrent disease, particularly associated with HCV infection. Also, morbidity related to side effects clearly mandates more rational use of IS in order to minimize the impact of diabetes, renal insufficiency, and atherosclerotic disease.

Induction therapy with anti-CD25 antibodies appears to be a worthwhile method to achieve effective early immunosuppression using either low-dose CNI or corticosteroid-free regimens. The potential for postoperative infections or IS side effects may be reduced with CNI weaning or replacement, leading to decreased risk of nephrotoxicity and neurotoxicity. This can be achieved with MMF or sirolimus, but the latter appears more effective for complete CNI avoidance when desirable. We also believe that modern IS protocols need only include very moderate or short-term use of corticosteroids, if any at all, as this can now be achieved using similar strategies to those used for CNI avoidance post-liver transplantation. We now see more liver recipients with a functioning graft dying of factors in common with the general population: heart disease and cancer. Tailored immunosuppression can help achieve the goal of reducing these risks. Sirolimus may prove useful in specific patients transplanted for hepatocellular carcinoma and is also a good candidate to reduce the risk of long-term cancer in the general transplant recipient population. Finally, newer drugs such as belatacept (LEA29Y) may replace more toxic immunosuppressive compounds to help minimize IS side effects.

With such approaches, regimens may be tailored to the comorbidities of recipients with the potential to achieve both improved survival and quality of life and reduced short- and long-term morbidity. As an ever-increasing range of anti-rejection agents are made available to clinicians, risk assessment and individualization of immunosuppressive treatment should continue to gain importance in clinical practice.

REFERENCES

1. Tippner C, Nashan B, Hoshino K, et al. Clinical and subclinical acute rejection early after liver transplantation: Contributing factors and relevance for the long-term course. *Transplantation* 2001; 72: 1122–8.
2. Knight RJ, Burrows L, Bodian C. The influence of acute rejection on long-term renal allograft survival: A comparison of living and cadaveric donor transplantation. *Transplantation* 2001; 72: 69–76.
3. Neuhaus P, Clavien P-A, Kittur D, et al. Improved treatment response with basiliximab immunoprophylaxis after liver transplantation: Results from a double-blind randomized placebo-controlled trial. *Liver Transpl* 2002; 8(2):132–42.
4. Emre S, Gondolesi G, Polat K, et al. Use of daclizumab as initial immunosuppression in liver transplant recipients with impaired renal function. *Liver Transpl* 2001; 7(3): 220–5.

5. Calmus Y, Scheele JR, Gonzalez-Pinto I, et al. Immunoprophylaxis with basiliximab, a chimeric anti-interleukin-2 receptor monoclonal antibody, in combination with azathioprine-containing triple therapy in liver transplant recipients. *Liver Transpl* 2002; 8(2): 123–31.

6. Koch M, Niemeyer G, Patel I, Light S, Nashan B. Pharmacokinetics, pharmacodynamics, and immunodynamics of daclizumab in a two-dose regimen in liver transplantation. *Transplantation* 2002; 73(10): 1640–6.

7. Ryan EA, Lakey JR, Paty BW, et al. Successful islet transplantation: Continued insulin reserve provides long-term glycemic control. *Diabetes* 2002; 51: 2148–57.

8. Washburn K, Speeg KV, Esterl R, et al. Steroid elimination 24 hours after liver transplantation using daclizumab, tacrolimus, and mycophenolate mofetil. *Transplantation* 2001; 72(10): 1675–9.

9. Boillot O, Mayer DA, Boudjema K, et al. Corticosteroid-free immunosuppression with tacrolimus following induction with daclizumab: A large randomized clinical study. *Liver Transpl* 2005; 11(1): 61–7.

10. Yoshida EM, Moratta PJ, Greig PD, et al. Evaluation of renal function in liver transplant recipients receiving daclizumab (Zenapax), mycophenolate mofetil, and a delayed, low-dose tacrolimus regimen vs. a standard-dose tacrolimus and mycophenolate mofetil regimen: A multicenter randomized clinical trial. *Liver Transpl* 2005; 11(9): 1064–72.

11. Eckhoff DE, McGuire B, Sellers M, et al. The safety and efficacy of two-dose daclizumab (Zenapax) induction therapy in liver transplant recipients. *Transplantation* 2000; 69(9): 1867–72.

12. Sellers MT, McGuire B, Haustein SV, Bynon JS, Hunt SL, Eckhoff DE. Two-dose daclizumab induction therapy in 209 liver transplants: A single-center analysis. *Transplantation* 2004; 78(8): 1212–7.

13. Yan LN, Wang W, Li B, et al. Single-dose daclizumab induction therapy in patients with liver transplantation. *World J Gastroenterol* 2003; 9(8): 1881–3.

14. Hirose R, Roberts JP, Quan D, et al. Experience with daclizumab in liver transplantation: Renal transplant dosing without calcineurin inhibitors is insufficient to prevent acute rejection in liver transplantation. *Transplantation* 2000; 69(2):307–11.

15. Pawarode A, Fine DM, Thuluvath PJ. Independent risk factors and natural history of renal dysfunction in liver transplant recipients. *Liver Transpl* 2003; 9: 741–7.

16. Nelson DR, Soldevila-Pico C, Reed A, et al. Anti-interleukin-2 receptor therapy in combination with mycophenolate mofetil is associated with more severe hepatitis C recurrence after liver transplantation. *Liver Transpl* 2001; 7(12): 1064–70.

17. Kato T, Yoshida H, Sadfar K, et al. Steroid-free induction and preemptive antiviral therapy for liver transplant recipients with hepatitis C: A preliminary report from a prospective randomized study. *Transpl Proc* 2005; 37(2): 1217–19.

18. Pham K, Kraft K, Thielke J, et al. Limited-dose daclizumab versus basiliximab: A comparison of cost and efficacy in preventing acute rejection. *Transpl Proc* 2005; 37(2): 899–902.

19. Amlot PL, Rawlings E, Fernando ON, et al. Prolonged action of a chimeric interleukin-2 receptor (CD25) monoclonal antibody used in cadaveric renal transplantation. *Transplantation* 1995; 60(7): 748–56.
20. Kovarik JM, Nashan B, Neuhaus P, et al. A population pharmacokinetic screen to identify demographic-clinical covariates of basiliximab in liver transplantation. *Clin Pharmacol Ther* 2001; 69(4): 201–9.
21. Kovarik J, Breidenbach T, Gerbeau C, Korn A, Schmidt AG, Hashan B. Disposition and immunodynamics of basiliximab in liver allograft recipients. *Clin Pharmacol Ther* 1998; 64(1): 66–72.
22. Aw MM, Taylor RM, Verma A, et al. Basiliximab (Simulect) for the treatment of steroid-resistant rejection in pediatric liver transplant recipients: A preliminary experience. *Transplantation* 2003; 75(6): 796–9.
23. Fernandes ML, Lee YM, Sutedja D, et al. Treatment of steroid-resistant acute liver transplant rejection with basiliximab. *Transpl Proc* 2005; 37(5): 2179–80.
24. Liu CL, Fan ST, Lo CM, et al. Interleukin-2 receptor antibody (basiliximab) for immunosuppressive induction therapy after liver transplantation: A protocol with early elimination of steroids and reduction of tacrolimus dosage. *Liver Transpl* 2004; 10(6): 728–33.
25. Filipponi F, Callea F, Salizzoni M, et al. Double-blind comparison of hepatitis C histological recurrence rate in HCV+ liver transplant recipients given basiliximab + steroids or basiliximab + placebo, in addition to cyclosporine and azathioprine. *Transplantation* 2004; 78(10): 1488–95.
26. Marcos A, Eghtesad B, Fung J, et al. Use of alemtuzumab and tacrolimus monotherapy for cadaveric liver transplantation: With particular reference to hepatitis C virus. *Transplantation* 2004; 78(7): 966–71.
27. Rebello PR, Hale G, Friend PJ, Cobbold SP, Waldmann H. Anti-globulin responses to rat and humanized CAMPATH-1 monoclonal antibody used to treat transplant rejection. *Transplantation* 1999; 68(9): 1417–20.
28. Watson CJ, Bradley JA, Friend PJ, et al. Alemtuzumab (Campath-1H) induction therapy in cadaveric kidney transplantation–Efficacy and safety at five years. *Am J Transpl* 2005; 5(6): 1347–53.
29. Knechtle SJ, Pirsch JD, Fechner J, et al. Campath-1H induction plus rapamycin monotherapy for renal transplantation: Results of a pilot study. *Am J Transpl* 2003; 3(6): 722–30.
30. Tzakis A, Tryphonopoulos P, Kato T, et al. Preliminary experience with alemtuzumab (Campath-1H) and low-dose tacrolimus immunosuppression in adult liver transplantation. *Transplantation* 2004; 77(8): 1209–14.
31. Weisner R, Sorrell M, Villamil F, and the International Liver Transplantation Society Panel. Report of the First International Liver Transplantation Society Expert Panel Consensus Conference on liver transplantation and hepatitis C. *Liver Transpl* 2003; 9(Suppl 3): S1–S9.
32. Jonas S, Rayes N, Neumann U, et al. De novo malignancies after liver transplantation using tacrolimus-based protocols or cyclosporin-based quadruple immunosuppression with an interleukin-2 receptor antibody or antithymocyte globulin. *Cancer* 1997; 80(6): 1141–50.
33. Vezina C, Kudelski A, Sehgal SN. Rapamycin (AY-22,989), a new antifungal antibiotic. I. Taxonomy of the producing streptomycete and isolation of the active principle. *J Antibiot* 1975; 28(10): 721–6.

34. Lai J-H, Tan T-H. CD28 signaling causes a sustained down-regulation of IkBa which can be prevented by the immunosuppressant rapamycin. *J Biol Chem* 1994; 269(48): 30077–80.

35. Yakupoglu YK, Kahan BD. Sirolimus: A current perspective. *Exp Clin Transpl* 2003; 1(1): 8–18.

36. Wiesner R, Klintmalm G, McDiarmid S, Rapamune Liver Transplant Study Group. Sirolimus immunotherapy results in reduced rates of acute rejection in de novo orthotopic liver transplant recipients. *Am J Transpl* 2002; 2: 464.

37. Wiesner R. The safety and efficacy of sirolimus and low-dose tacrolimus versus tacrolimus in de novo orthotopic liver transplant recipients. Results from a pilot study. *Hepatology* 2002; 36:280A.

38. Trotter JF, Wachs M, Bak T, et al. Liver transplantation using sirolimus and minimal corticoids (3-day taper). *Liver Transpl* 2001; 7(4): 343–51.

39. Dunkelberg JC, Trotter JF, Wachs M, et al. Sirolimus as primary immunosuppression in liver transplantation is not associated with hepatic artery or wound complications. *Liver Transpl* 2003; 9(5): 463–8.

40. McAlister VC, Peltekian KM, Malatjalian DA, et al. Orthotopic liver transplantation using low-dose tacrolimus and sirolimus. *Liver Transpl* 2001; 7: 701–8.

41. Kneteman N, Oberholzer J, Al Saghier M, et al. Sirolimus-based immunosuppression for liver transplantation in the presence of extended criteria for hepatocellular carcinoma. *Liver Transpl* 2004; 10(10): 1301–11.

42. Montalbano M, Neff GW, Yamashiki N, et al. A retrospective review of liver transplant patients treated with sirolimus from a single center: An analysis of sirolimus-related complications. *Transplantation* 2004; 78: 264–8.

43. Trotter JF, Wachs M, Trouillot T, et al. Dyslipidemia during sirolimus therapy in liver transplant recipients occurs with concomitant cyclosporin but not tacrolimus. *Liver Transpl* 2001; 7(5): 401–8.

44. Ryan EA, Paty BW, Senior PA, et al. Five-year follow-up after clinical islet transplantation. *Diabetes* 2005: 54(7): 2060–9.

45. Kauffman HM, Cherikh WS, Cheng Y, Hanto DW, Kahan BD. Maintenance immunosuppression with target-of-rapamycin inhibitors is associated with a reduced incidence of de novo malignancies. *Am J Transpl* 2005; 80: 883–9.

46. Guba M, Graeb C, Jauch KW, Geissler EK. Pro- and anti-cancer effects of immunosuppressive agents used in organ transplantation. *Transplantation* 2004; 77(12): 1777–82.

47. Majno P, Giostra E, Mentha G, Geneva Liver Cancer Study Group. Is there a customised immunosuppression regimen for patients transplanted with hepatocellular carcinoma? *J Hepatol* 2005; 43(4): 577–84.

48. Eng CP, Sehgal SN, Vezina C. Activity of rapamycin (AY-22,989) against transplanted tumors. *J Antibiot* 1984; 37(10): 1231–7.

49. Guba M, von Breitenbuch P, Steinbauer M, et al. Rapamycin inhibits primary and metastatic tumor growth by antiangiogenesis: Involvement of vascular endothelial growth factor. *Nat Med* 2002; 8(2): 128–35.

50. Guba M, Yezhelyev M, Eichhorn ME, et al. Rapamycin induces tumor-specific thrombosis via tissue factor in the presence of VEGF. *Blood* 2005; 105: 4463–9.

51. Mazzaferro V, Regalia E, Doci R, et al. Liver transplantation for the treatment of small hepatocellular carcinomas in patients with cirrhosis. *N Engl J Med* 1996; 334(11): 693–9.

52. Vivarelli M, Bellusci R, Cucchetti A, et al. Low recurrence rate of hepatocellular carcinoma after liver transplantation: Better patient selection or lower immunosuppression? *Transplantation* 2002; 74(12): 1746–51.

53. Mulay AV, Hussain N, Fergusson D, Knoll GA. Calcineurin inhibitor withdrawal from sirolimus-based therapy in kidney transplantation: A systematic review of randomized trials. *Am J Transpl* 2005; 5(7): 1748–56.

54. Neff GW, Montalbano M, Slapak-Green G, et al. Sirolimus therapy in orthotopic liver transplant recipients with calcineurin inhibitor related chronic renal insufficiency. *Transpl Proc* 2003; 35(8):3029–31.

55. Fairbanks KD, Eustace JA, Fine A, Thuluvath PJ. Renal function improves in liver transplant recipient when switched from a calcineurin inhibitor to sirolimus. *Liver Transpl* 2003; 9(10):1079–85.

56. Letavernier E, Pe'raldi MN, Pariente A, Morelon E, Legendre C. Proteinuria following a switch from calcineurin inhibitors to sirolimus. *Transplantation* 2005; 80(9):1198–203.

57. Andres A, Toso C, Morel P, et al. Impairment of renal function after islet transplant alone or islet-after-kidney transplantation using a sirolimus/tacrolimus-based immunosuppression regimen. *Transpl Int* 2005; 18(11):1226–30.

58. Nashan B, Curtis J, Ponticelli C, et al. Everolimus and reduced-exposure cyclosporin in de novo renal-transplant recipients: A three-year phase II, randomized, multicenter, open-label study. *Transplantation* 2004; 78(9):1332–40.

59. Lorber MI, Mulgaonkar S, Butt KM, et al. Everolimus versus mycophenolate mofetil in the prevention of rejection in de novo renal transplant recipients: A 3-year randomized, multicenter, phase III study. *Transplantation* 2005; 80(2): 244–52.

60. Brinkmann V. FTY720: Mechanism of action and potential benefit in organ transplantation. *Yonsei Med J* 2004; 45(6):991–7.

61. Kahan BD, Karlix JL, Ferguson RM, Leichtman AB, Mulgaonkar S, Gonwa TA. Pharmacodynamics, pharmacokinetics, and safety of mutiple doses of FTY720 in stable renal transplant patients: A multicenter, randomized, placebo-controlled, phase I study. *Transplantation* 2003; 76:1079–84.

62. Tedesco-Silva H, Mourad G, Kahan BD, et al. FTY720, a novel immunomodulator: Efficacy and safety results from the first phase 2A study in de novo renal transplantation. *Transplantation* 2005; 79(11):1553–60.

63. Furukawa H, Susuki T, Jin MB, et al. Prolongation of canine liver allograft survival by a novel immunosuppressant, FTY720: Effect of monotherapy and combined treatment with conventional drugs. *Transplantation* 2000; 69(2): 235–41.

64. Anselmo DM, Amersi FF, Shen XD, et al. FTY720 pretreatment reduces warm hepatic ischemia reperfusion injury through inhibition of T-lymphocyte infiltration. *Am J Transpl* 2002; 2(9):843–9.

65. Fitzsimmons WE, First MR. FK778, a synthetic malononitrilamide. *Yonsei Med J* 2004; 45(6):1132–5.

66. Vanrenterghem Y, van Hooff JP, Klinger M, et al. The effects of FK778 in combination with tacrolimus and steroids–A phase II multicenter study in renal transplant patients. *Transplantation* 2004; 78:9–14.

67. Satoshi Y, Toyokazu O, Keiichi Y, et al. FK778 and FK506 combination therapy to control acute rejection after rat liver allotransplantation. *Transplantation* 2004; 78(11):1618–25.

68. Kremer J, Westhovens R, Leon M, et al. Treatment of rheumatoid arthritis by selective inhibition of T-cell activation with fusion protein CTLA4Ig. *N Engl J Med* 2003; 349(20):1907–15.

69. Larsen C, Pearson T, Adams A, et al. Rational development of LEA29Y (belatacept), a high-affinity variant of CTLA4-Ig with potent immunosuppressive properties. *Am J Transpl* 2005; 5:443–53.

70. Vincenti F, Larsen C, Durrbach A, et al. Costimulation blockade with belatacept in renal transplantation. *N Engl J Med* 2005; 353:770–81.

71. Bartlett AS, McCall JL, Ameratunga R, et al. Costimulatory blockade prevents early rejection, promotes lymphocyte apoptosis, and inhibits the upregulation of intragraft interleukin-6 in an orthotopic liver transplant model in the rat. *Liver Transpl* 2002; 8(5):458–68.

72. Marder B, Schroppel B, Lin M, et al. The impact of costimulatory molecule gene polymorphisms on clinical outcomes in liver transplantation. *Am J Transpl* 2003; 3:424–31.

73. Annual report of the U.S. organ procurement and transplantation network and the scientific registry of transplant recipients: Transplant data 1993–2002. 2003, HHS/HRSA.SPB/DOT; UNOS; URREA: Rockville, MD.

74. Berenguer M, Ferrell L, Watson J, et al. HCV-related fibrosis progression following liver transplantation: Increase in recent years. *J Hepatol* 2000; 32:673–84.

75. Ghobrial R, Steadman R, Gornbein J, et al. A 10-year experience of liver transplantation for hepatitis C: Analysis of factors determining outcome in over 500 patients. *Ann Surg* 2001; 234:384–93.

76. Bahra M, Neumann U, Jacob D, Langrehr J, Neuhaus P. Repeated steroid pulse therapies in HCV-positive liver recipients: Significant risk factor for HCV-related graft loss. *Transpl Proc* 2005; 37:1700–2.

77. Gane E, Naoumov N, Qian K, et al. A longituinal analysis of hepatitis C virus replication following liver transplantation. *Gastroenterology* 1996; 110:167–77.

78. Sheiner P, Schwartz M, Mor E, et al. Severe or multiple rejection episodes are associated with early recurrence of hepatitis C after orthotopic liver transplantation. *Hepatology* 1995; 21:30–4.

79. Rosen H, Shackleton C, Higa L, et al. Use of OKT3 is associated with early and severe recurrence of hepatitis C after liver transplantation. *Am J Gastroenterol* 1997; 92:1453–7.

80. Charlton M, Seaberg E. Impact of immunosuppression and acute rejection on recurrence of hepatitis C: Results of the National Institute of Diabetes and Digestive and Kidney Diseases Liver Transplantation Database. *Liver Transpl Surg* 1999; 5:S107–S114.

81. Wiesner R. A long-term comparison of tacrolimus (FK506) versus cyclosporine in liver transplantation: A report of the United States FK506 Study Group. *Transplantation* 1998; 66:493–9.

82. Eason J, Loss G, Blazek J, et al. Steroid-free liver transplantation using rabbit antithymocyte globulin induction: Results of a prospective randomized trial. *Liver Transpl* 2001; 7:693–7.

83. Kneteman N. Steroid-free immunosuppression: Balancing efficacy and toxicity. *Liver Transpl* 2001; 7:698–700.

84. Margarit C, Bilbao I, Castells L, et al. A prospective randomized trial comparing tacrolimus and steroids with tacrolimus monotherapy in liver transplantation: The impact on recurrence of hepatitis C. *Transplant Int* 2005; 18(12):1336–45.

85. Brillanti S, Vivarelli M, DeRuvo N, et al. Slowly tapering off steroids protects the graft against hepatitis C recurrence after liver transplantation. *Liver Transpl* 2002; 8:884–8.

86. Lake J. The role of immunosuppression in recurrence of hepatitis C. *Liver Transpl* 2003; 9(Suppl 3):S63–S66.

87. Fasola C, Netto G, Christensen L, et al. Lower incidences of early hepatitis C RNA levels and HCV recurrence post liver transplantation in patients induced with mycopenolate mofetil: A high-dose benefit. *Liver Transpl* 2002; 8:C52A.

88. Wiesner R, Shorr J, Steffen B, Chu A, Gordon R, Lake J. Mycophenolate mofetil combination therapy improves long-term outcomes after liver transplantation in patients with and without hepatitis C. *Liver Transpl* 2005; 11(7):750–9.

89. Jain A, Kashyap R, Demetris A, Eghstesad B, Pokharna R, Fung JJ. A prospective randomized trial of mycophenolate mofetil in liver transplant recipients with hepatitis C. *Liver Transpl* 2002; 8(1):47–9.

90. Samonakis D, Triantos C, Thalheimer U, et al. Immunosuppression and donor age with respect to severity of HCV recurrence after liver transplantation. *Liver Transpl* 2005; 11(4):386–95.

91. Watashi K, HijikataM, Hosaka M, Yamaji M, Shijotohno K. Cyclosporin A suppresses replication of hepatitis C virus genome in cultured hepatocytes. *Hepatology* 2003; 38:1282–8.

92. Nakagawa M, Sakamoto N, Enomoto N, et al. Specific inhibition of hepatitis C virus replication by cyclosporin A. *Biochem Biophys Res Commun* 2004; 313:42–7.

93. Watashi K, Ishii N, Hijikata M, Inoue D, et al. Cyclophilin B is a functional regulator of hepatitis C virus RNA polymerase. *Mol Cell* 2005; 19:111–22.

94. Nakagawa M, Sakamoto N, Tanabe Y, et al. Suppression of hepatitis C virus replication by cyclosporin A is mediated by blockade of cyclophilins. *Gastroenterology* 2005; 129:1031–41.

95. Inoue K, Sekiyama K, Yamada M, Watanabe T, et al. Combined interferon alpha 2b and cyclosporin A in the treatment of chronic hepatitis C: Controlled trial. *J Gastroenterol* 2003; 38:567–72.

96. Inoue K, Yoshiba M. Interferon combined with cyclosporin treatment as an effective countermeasure against hepatitis C recurrence in liver transplant patients with end-stage hepatitis C virus related disease. *Transpl Proc* 2005; 37:1233–4.

97. Akiyama H, Yoshimaga H, Tanaka T, et al. Effects of cyclosporin A on hepatitis C virus infection in bone marrow transplant patients. *Bone Marrow Transpl* 1997; 20:993–5.

98. Firpi FJ, Zhu H, Morelli G, et al. Cyclosporine suppresses hepatitis C virus *in vitro* and increases the chance of a sustained virological response after liver transplantation. *Liver Transpl* 2006;12:51–7.

99. Zervos X, Weppler D, Gragulidis G, et al. Comparison of tacrolimus with microemulsion cyclosporin as primary immunosuppression in hepatitis C patients after liver transplantation. *Transplantation* 1998; 65:1044–6.

100. Martin P, Busutill R, Crippin J, Klintmalm G, Fitzsimmons W, Uleman C. Impact of tacrolimus versus cyclosporin in hepatitis C virus-infected recipients on recurrent hepatitis: A prospective, randomized trial. *Liver Transpl* 2004; 10(10):1258–62.
101. Levy G, Villamil F, Samuel D, et al. LIS2T Study Group. Results of LIS2T, a multicenter, randomized study comparing cyclosporine microemulsion with C2 monitoring and tacrolimus with C0 monitoring in de novo liver transplantation. *Transplantation* 2004; 77(11):1632–8.
102. Samonakis D, Cholongitas E, Triantos C, et al. Sustained, spontaneous disappearance of serum HCV-RNA under immunosuppression after liver transplantation for HCV cirrhosis. *Liver Transpl* 2005; 43(6):1091–3.
103. Liermann-Garcia RF, Evangelista-Garcia C, McMaster P, Neuberger J. Transplantation for primary biliary cirrhosis: Retrospective analysis of 400 patients in a single center. *Hepatology* 2001; 33:22–7.
104. Lohmann V, Korner F, Koch J, Herian U, Theilmann L, Bartenschlager R. Replication of subgenomic hepatitis C virus RNAs in a hepatoma cell line. *Science* 1999; 285(5424):110–3.
105. Lindenbach BD, Evans MJ, Snyder AJ, et al. Complete replication of hepatitis C virus in cell culture. *Science* 2005; 309(5734):623–6.
106. Wakita T, Pietschmann T, Kato T, et al. Production of infectious hepatitis C virus in tissue culture from a cloned viral genome. *Nat Med* 2005; 11(7):791–6.
107. Mercer DF, Schiller DE, Elliott JF, et al. Hepatitis C virus replication in mice with chimeric human livers. *Nat Med* 2001; 7(8):927–33.

3

Pre- and Posttransplant Management of Hepatitis C

Norah A. Terrault, MD, MPH and Mario G. Pessoa

CONTENTS

Abstract

Hepatitis C is the most common indication for liver transplantation in the United States. Reinfection is a universal occurrence in patients who are transplanted with viremia, and recurrent hepatitis results in higher rates of graft and patient loss compared to other indications for transplantation. The most important factors that predict poor transplant outcome are advanced donor age and treatment of acute rejection. Therapy may be given prior to transplantation to eradicate virus and prevent recurrent disease. Alternatively, posttransplantation therapy can be administered prior to the development of overt clinical

From: *Clinical Gastroenterology: Liver Transplantation: Challenging
Controversies and Topics*
Edited by: G. T. Everson and J. F. Trotter, DOI: 10.1007/978-1-60327-028-1_3,
© Humana Press, Totowa, NJ

disease (early or preemptive therapy) or delayed until histological progression is evident. However, posttransplantation therapy with interferon and ribavirin is problematic due to a high incidence of treatment complications and low sustained virologic response rate. New therapies that are more uniformly effective and better tolerated are needed to improve virologic response rates and ultimately reduce the rates of cirrhosis and graft loss.

Key Words: Immunosuppression; Cirrhosis; Pegylated interferon; Ribavirin; Decompensated; Preemptive

INTRODUCTION

End-stage liver disease secondary to the hepatitis C virus (HCV) is the leading indication for liver transplantation in most transplant centers in the North America and Western Europe. Long-term graft and patient survival in HCV-infected transplant recipients is lower than in patients transplanted for other indications, with a 23% higher rate of death and a 30% higher rate of graft loss five years' posttransplantation (1). The higher rate of patient and graft loss reflects the complications of recurrent disease. Recurrent HCV cirrhosis accounts for up to 36% of deaths in patients transplanted for HCV (2).

Graft reinfection with HCV is essentially universal in persons who are viremic pretransplantation (3). There is an accelerated rate of disease progression after liver transplantation, with an estimated median time from transplantation to cirrhosis of 8 to 12 years (4–8). Once cirrhosis is present, up to 42% develop liver decompensation within one year (9). Cholestatic hepatitis, the most severe and aggressive form of recurrent HCV infection, develops in up to 5–10% of patients (10, 11).

FACTORS INFLUENCING THE NATURAL HISTORY OF POSTTRANSPLANT HCV DISEASE

Several factors have been found to be associated with higher rates of cirrhosis or progressive fibrosis (Table 1), but the factors most consistent across multiple studies are older donor age, cytomegalovirus (CMV) infection, and treatment of acute rejection (use of steroid pulses or antilymphocyte therapies such as OKT3) (7, 12–17). The relative risk for graft loss for transplant recipients who received a organ from a donor aged 41–50, 51–60, and >60 years of age was 1.67 (95% CI: 1.34–2.09), 1.86 (1.48–2.34), and 2.21 (1.73–2.81) times greater than that with a donor <40 years of age (15). Treatment of acute rejection

Table 1
Factors Associated with HCV Disease Severity

Category	Factor Linked with More Severe Disease
Donor factors	Older donor age Longer cold ischemia time Longer warm ischemia time
Recipient factors	Posttransplant diabetes mellitus HCV genotype 1
Viral factors	High HCV viral load at transplant CMV infection
Transplant-related factors	Treated acute rejection OKT3 use Corticosteroid boluses Short time to recurrence

with steroid pulses or antilymphocyte therapies has been associated with a higher risk of cirrhosis and fibrosis progression (7, 16, 17). CMV infection has a pro-fibrogenic effect on HCV disease, but the underlying mechanism is uncertain (14, 17). Higher pretransplant HCV RNA levels have been linked with more severe disease and reduced survival in some studies (13, 18).

Other factors of potential importance, identified less consistently across studies, include cold and warm ischemia times, posttransplant diabetes, early recurrence of HCV, living donor liver transplantation, HCV genotype, and donor–recipient HLA matching (19, 20). Genotype 1b has been associated with more progressive HCV disease in some but not all studies. Living donor liver transplant recipients have a higher rate of graft loss than deceased donor transplant recipients, which appears to be related to the transplant center's experience with living donor transplantation (21). However, whether the type of donor influences HCV fibrosis progression is unclear, as studies addressing this issue have reported very different results. Garcia-Retortillo et al. reported a two-year probability of developing cirrhosis of 22% in deceased donor recipients versus 45% in living donor recipients ($p = 0.019$) (22). Shiffman et al., in contrast, found a threefold lower risk of advanced fibrosis (12% vs. 39%, respectively) in living donor recipients compared to deceased donor recipients after 36 months of follow-up (23).

Immunosuppression is undoubtedly an important factor in the natural history of HCV following transplantation. The optimal immunosuppressive regimen, however, remains to be defined. Cyclosporine has HCV-suppressive effects *in vitro* (24), but in longitudinal studies evaluating outcomes in recipients receiving tacrolimus-based therapy versus cyclosporine-based therapy, no differences in HCV disease severity or risk of cirrhosis were shown (25–29). Mycophenolate mofetil has no consistent effect, either positive or negative, on HCV histology and risk of cirrhosis (30–32). Steroid-free immunosuppression and regimens of rapid steroid tapering appear to have a beneficial effect on metabolic complications, but no clear benefit on HCV disease progression. HCV RNA levels are significantly different in steroid-containing versus steroid-sparing regimes. Since steroid-free regimens frequently use anti-interleukin-2 receptor antibodies or lymphocyte-depleting agents also, the independent contribution of steroid elimination and use of lymphocyte-depleting drugs is difficult to discern (33, 34). Late withdrawal of steroids has also been proposed to be protective against recurrent HCV. Results are again inconsistent across studies (28, 35, 36).

Given the lack of clear benefits of one regimen over another, no specific immunosuppressive combination can be advocated on an empirical basis. Studies comparing combinations of immunosuppressive agents of differing "potency" suggest less immunosuppression is better for HCV-infected patients (28, 37, 38). Additionally, withdrawal of immunosuppression in stable patients led to improved histology in one study (39). These results require confirmation but are in keeping with the "less-is-better" concept of immunosuppression in HCV-infected patients.

TREATMENT STRATEGIES FOR PATIENTS WITH CHRONIC HCV UNDERGOING LIVER TRANSPLANTATION

To *prevent* recurrent HCV disease, treatment must be given prior to transplantation, with the goal of achieving viral eradication or suppression prior to transplantation. Achievement of a sustained virologic response prior to transplantation prevents recurrent HCV posttransplantation (40, 41). Pretransplant therapy using pegylated interferon (peg-IFN) and ribavirin (RBV) is an option for selected patients. Treatment is limited by poor tolerability of current therapies in patients with decompensated cirrhosis. Prophylactic therapies for HCV, if available, would be started at or near the time of transplantation and continued post-transplantation for limited or prolonged periods, as is done with HBV therapies in liver transplant patients. At the present time, there are no effective prophylactic therapies (42, 43).

Since the majority of patients are viremic at the time of transplantation and develop recurrent disease, the focus of HCV management remains in the posttransplant period. Combination pegylated interferon and ribavirin is the treatment of choice for recurrent HCV disease. In the posttransplant setting, the primary goal of therapy is to prevent graft loss due to recurrent HCV. Achievement of a sustained virological response (SVR) is associated with improvements or stabilization of histological disease in the majority of patients. The optimal management of nonresponders to antiviral therapy has not been defined.

In order to identify patients with progressive histological disease who warrant consideration of treatment, most transplant centers perform protocol liver biopsies on a yearly basis (44). The diagnosis of recurrent HCV disease can be difficult to distinguish from acute cellular rejection and recurrent HCV disease (45, 46) and requires an experienced liver pathologist. Misdiagnosis has important implications, as treatment of misdiagnosed acute rejection with increased immunosuppression has detrimental effects on HCV disease progression, and missed acute rejection treated with interferon has detrimental effects on rejection severity.

Pretransplant Management of Chronic HCV

For patients with decompensated cirrhosis, anti-HCV treatment is generally considered a contraindication. However, as highlighted previously, the rationale for treatment of HCV prior to transplantation is that viral eradication prior to organ implantation will prevent or reduce the risk of recurrent infection posttransplantation and therefore improve graft and patient survival. Several recent studies have examined the safety and efficacy of antiviral therapy in patients awaiting transplantation. These studies suggest this treatment strategy may be applicable to a selected group of transplant candidates, but the efficacy of antiviral therapy is diminished compared to compensated patients with chronic HCV patients, and the frequency of side effects is increased (40, 41, 47).

The largest study of HCV treatment of decompensated cirrhotics used a low-ascending dose regimen (LADR) to maximize safety. A total of 124 patients with advanced liver disease were treated with starting doses of non-pegylated IFN 1.5 MU thrice weekly or peg-IFN (0.5 ug/kg peg-IFN-alpha-2b or 90 ug peg-IFN-alpha-2a) and ribavirin 600 mg daily and increasing in stepwise fashion to the standard target doses of IFN (3 MU thrice weekly) or peg-IFN (1.5 ug/kg peg-IFN-alpha-2b and 180 ug peg-IFN-alpha-2a) and ribavirin 1,000–1,200 mg daily (40). The majority had Child's class B and C cirrhosis (55%), with a mean Model for End-stage Liver Disease (MELD) score of 8.4, 11.1, and 16.8 for those with Child's A, B, and C cirrhosis, respectively. The end-of-treatment virologic response (EOTVR) rate was 46%, and the overall rate of sustained virological response was 22%. Twenty-three nonresponders and relapsers of non-pegylated IFN and ribavirin were retreated with peg-IFN and ribavirin, and three (13%) became HCV RNA–negative. Genotype was an important determinant of response: The SVR rate was 50% among patients with HCV genotype 2 or 3 and 13% among patients with genotype 1. Patients who had an SVR before transplantation did not experience recurrent disease after transplantation. Of interest, six of eight patients who were HCV RNA-negative but still on treatment at the time of transplantation remained HCV RNA-negative posttransplantation. In contrast, all the viremic nonresponders and relapsers who underwent transplantation developed recurrent HCV infection. Adverse events required discontinuation of therapy in 20% of patients. Liver-related complications occurred in 12% of patients.

In another study examining the efficacy of an on-treatment response in reducing the risk of recurrent HCV, 30 patients with HCV cirrhosis awaiting liver transplantation (50% Child's class B and C) were treated with IFN 3 MU daily and ribavirin 800 mg daily for a median of 12 weeks (41). Among patients achieving SVR before transplantation, none had HCV recurrence posttransplantation. Of nine patients with an on-treatment virologic response, six remained HCV RNA-negative following transplantation after a median follow-up of 46 weeks. Discontinuation of therapy prematurely due to side effects was seen in 20% of treated patients, and dose reductions were necessary in 63% of patients despite the use of filgrastim and erythropoietin.

A third study evaluating the efficacy of IFN-based therapy in patients with more advanced liver disease highlights the serious side effects that occur with treatment, especially those with more advanced decompensation (47). In this randomized study, 15 UNOS status 2b liver transplant candidates (all Child's class B or C; 73% genotype 1) were treated with either IFN-alpha-2b 1 MU daily, IFN-alpha-2b 3 MU thrice weekly, or IFN-alpha-2b 1 MU daily plus ribavirin 400 mg twice daily. Growth factors were not used in this study. Five of 15 patients (33%) achieved EOTVR; two were transplanted, and both developed recurrent HCV infection. Thirteen of 15 patients experienced adverse events; the majority were graded as severe and the study was terminated early due to the frequency of adverse events. The authors concluded that patients with advanced liver disease are not candidates for antiviral therapy.

In summary, these studies demonstrate that attainment of SVR prior to transplantation can prevent recurrent HCV posttransplantation. Additionally, a proportion (>50%) of those with an on-treatment response (HCV RNA-negative) will remain virus-free posttransplantation. However, the tolerability of these drugs in patients with advanced decompensated liver disease is limited, and life-threatening complications can occur. Therefore, at the present time, the routine treatment of patients with decompensated cirrhosis cannot be recommended outside clinical trials. Given the frequency of complications, treatment should be provided only at experienced centers and to patients listed and ready for liver transplantation and only after a detailed discussion of risks and benefits with the patient.

Posttransplant Management of the Patient with Chronic HCV

There are two approaches to treatment of recurrent HCV infection posttransplantation: Antiviral treatment can be administered prior to the development of overt clinical disease (early or preemptive therapy) or delayed until histological progression is evident. The majority of studies have treated patients only when histological disease is moderate to severe and typically only when fibrosis is present. The reversibility of fibrosis may be dependent upon the severity of disease at the onset of treatment.

The only drugs currently available for the treatment of recurrent disease in transplant recipients are interferon (non-pegylated and pegylated forms) and ribavirin. Not surprisingly, the effectiveness of antiviral therapy is diminished in liver transplant recipients. Several factors contribute, including a high prevalence of genotype 1 and high baseline HCV RNA levels, a higher rate of dose reductions due to side effects especially cytopenias, and immunosuppressant effects of concurrent antirejection medications.

Preemptive Treatment of Recurrent HCV Infection

The rationale for treating HCV in the early posttransplant period originates from the recognition of the higher rates of SVR in HCV-infected nontransplant patients who have a low HCV viral load and less advanced fibrosis at baseline. In the early posttransplant period, viral loads are initially low and increase variably to reach peak values within three months of transplantation. Fibrosis is rare in the early posttransplant period, but approximately 50% of patients have at least early fibrosis at one year posttransplantation. However, the cons of treatment in the first weeks posttransplantation include the potentially detrimental effects of higher doses of immunosuppression on response rates, the more limited tolerability of therapy in recently transplanted patients, and the use of interferon when the risk of acute rejection is highest (first three months posttransplantation).

Preemptive anti-HCV treatment has been used with variable success and tolerability (Table 2). Earlier studies of IFN monotherapy achieved EOTVR in only 0–17% of treated patients and SVRs were not seen (48, 49). A recent randomized trial of peg-IFN 180 mcg/weekly monotherapy for 48 weeks, beginning 3 weeks after transplantation, achieved an SVR in only 8% of treated patients (50). Treated patients had significantly lower HCV RNA levels and better histological profiles than untreated patients at the end of the follow-up. Fibrosis scores improved or stabilized in 23 (88%) treated patients compared to only 11 (38%) untreated patients. The incidence of acute rejection was similar in the treated and untreated groups (12% vs. 21%). Shergill et al. compared preemptive IFN or peg-IFN monotherapy versus combination therapy with IFN or peg-IFN plus ribavirin (51). Patients were randomized within two to six weeks of transplantation to IFN-alpha-2b or peg-IFN-alpha-2b (3 MU thrice weekly or 1.5 mcg/kg weekly) versus IFN or peg-IFN plus RBV (600 mg increased to 1,0001–200 mg daily) for a total of 48 weeks. Dose reductions were required in 85% of patients, and early discontinuation of therapy was required in 37% despite the use of growth factors. EOTVR and SVR occurred in only 14% and 9%, respectively.

In contrast to the low SVR rates reported in the U.S. studies, Sugawara et al. reported an SVR rate of 39% among 23 HCV-infected live donor recipients treated with IFN 3 MU thrice weekly and RBV 400 mg daily begun within one month posttransplantation and continued for 48 weeks (52). Histological benefits were evident with lower histology activity index (HAI) scores in treated compared to untreated patients. However, dose reductions or early discontinuation of therapy occurred in 57% of patients. Mazzaferro et al. also reported a higher SVR rate than in U.S. studies, with 33% of treated patients achieving SVR with 12 months of IFN plus ribavirin (53), with a 100% SVR rate in those with genotype 2 and 20% SVR in genotype 1 patients.

In summary, preemptive therapy using combined IFN and ribavirin results in an SVR of 9–39%, with the highest responses in patients with non-genotype 1 infection and living donor recipients. Dose modifications are frequent and likely contribute to the low SVR rates. Mild histological disease was reported in the majority of patients treated with preemptive therapy, suggesting disease-modulating effects, but controlled studies are lacking. Responders have less severe histological

Table 2
Studies of Posttransplant Preemptive HCV Treatment[*]

Study	Regimen (No. of Patients)	Duration	Virologic Response	Histologic Response	Dose Reduction Discontinuation
Mazzaferro, 2004 (53)	IFN and RBV (N = 36)	12 mo	SVR: 33% Genotype 1: 20% Genotype 2: 100%	Improved Ishak score in responders (1.7) compared to nonresponders (3.3) at treatment end	25% dose reductions; no discontinuations
Sugawara, 2004 (52)	IFN and RBV (N = 23) All live donor LT recipients	12 mo	SVR: 39%	Improved HAI score at 1 year in treated patients	Dose modification or discontinuation in 57%
Shergill, 2005 (51)	(1) IFN or peg-IFN (N = 22) (2) IFN or peg-IFN plus RBV (N = 22)	48 wk	SVR: (1) 2.5% (2) 18%	70% stage 0 and 20% stage 1 at end of treatment	Dose reduction in 85% and early d/c in 37%

[*]IFN = interferon; LT = liver transplantation; RBV = ribavirin; SVR = sustained virologic response (undetectable HCV RNA six months after completion of therapy); HAI = histology activity index.

disease than nonresponders. At the present time, it is unclear whether preemptive therapy offers any benefits over treatment delayed until histological disease is present. A multicenter study comparing preemptive versus delayed treatment is underway and results are awaited. Clearly, the availability of more effective and better-tolerated antiviral agents would make preemptive therapy a more attractive treatment strategy.

Treatment of Posttransplant HCV Disease

Most clinicians wait until there is histological evidence of recurrent HCV disease before initiating treatment. Controlled trials on antiviral therapy are limited; most of the available studies are single-center and uncontrolled (54). Monotherapy with either interferon or pegylated interferon has shown low SVR rates (0–12%) (50, 55, 56). Combination therapy with interferon and ribavirin yields higher SVR rates, ranging from 13–30% (57–64) (Table 3). In the only controlled study of combination therapy, 28 patients were treated with recurrent HCV with IFN 3 MU thrice weekly and ribavirin 800–1,000 mg daily for 48 weeks and compared with 24 untreated controls (60). The SVR rate was in 21% of treated patients versus 0% in controls. In this study, there was no significant difference in histology in treated and untreated patients at six months posttreatment. Most uncontrolled studies comparing histology prior to and posttreatment report improvements in necroinflammatory scores in the majority, but improvements in fibrosis scores are seen less consistently (57–64).

Combined pegylated interferon and ribavirin appears to be the most effective therapy, although prospective studies comparing pegylated and non-pegylated IFN in combination with ribavirin have not been done. The majority of the studies have used pegylated IFN-alpha-2b at doses ranging from 0.5 to 1.5 ug/kg weekly in combination with ribavirin (Table 3). The majority of patients were infected with genotype 1 infection (90% or greater). SVR rates range from 26–45% (median 30%) in studies with at least 20 patients (62, 65–67). These SVR rates are generally higher than those reported for non-pegylated interferon plus ribavirin (13–30%, median 26%), supporting the conclusion that pegylated interferon plus ribavirin is the treatment of choice in posttransplant patients.

The study by Castells et al. (66) differs from the other peg-IFN plus ribavirin studies in that patient population was 24 patients with genotype 1b infection presenting in the acute phase of HCV recurrence. Of 23 patients who reached week 24 of treatment, 8 (35%) achieved an SVR. Surprisingly, no patients dropped out because of adverse effects,

Table 3
Studies of Posttransplant Recurrent HCV Treatment*

Reference	N	Treatment Regimen	SVR Rate	Dose Reduction or Discontinuation
Non-Pegylated Interferon Plus Ribavirin				
Samuel 2003 (60)	52	(1) IFN 3 MU TIW and RBV 800–1,200 mg QD (28) × 12 mo (2) No treatment (24)	21% vs. 0% in controls	43% early d/c
Firpi, 2002 (58)	54	IFN 3 MU TIW and RBV 800–1,000 mg QD × 12 mo	30%	72% dose reduction
Giostra, 2004 (57)	31	RBV 10 mg/kg QD × 12 wk; then RBV and IFN 3 MU TIW up to 60 wk	29%	77% early d/c or dose reductions
Bizollon, 2003 (61)	54	IFN 3 MU TIW and RBV 1,000 mg QD × 6 mo; then RBV × 12 mo	26%	11% early d/c of RBV
Berenguer, 2004 (64)	24	IFN 1.5–3 MU TIW and RBV 600–1,200 mg QD × 12 mo; then RBV × 6 mo	12.5%	29% early d/c 88% dose reduction
Dumortier, 2004 (62)	20	Peg-IFN-alpha-2b 0.5–1 mcg/kg/wk and RBV 400–1,200 mg QD × 12 mo	45%	20% early d/c Dose reduction: 30% IFN 64% RBV

Table 3
Studies of Posttransplant Recurrent HCV Treatment*

Reference	N	Treatment Regimen	SVR Rate	Dose Reduction or Discontinuation
Pegylated Interferon and Ribavirin				
Castells, 2005 (66)	24	Peg-IFN-alpha-2b 1.5 μg/kg/wk plus RBV 600 mg/day for 24–48 wk	35%	Discontinuation in 12.5% Dose reductions for anemia in 58%
Rodriguez-Luna, 2004 (67)	37	Peg-IFN-alpha-2b 0.5–1.5 μg/kg/wk plus RBV 400–1,000 mg/day for ≥48 wk	26%	37% early d/c
Oton, 2006 (65)	55	Peg-IFN-alpha-2b 1.5 ug/kg/wk (N = 51) or Peg-IFN-alpha-2a 180 ug (N = 4) plus ribavirin (>11 mg/kg/day)	44%	29% early d/c

*Limited to studies of at least 20 treated patients.

IFN = interferon; RBV = ribavirin; MU = million units; QD = once daily; TIW = thrice weekly; d/c = discontinuation; EOTVR = end of treatment virologic response (undetectable HCV RNA by PCR); SVR = sustained virologic response (undetectable HCV RNA six months after completion of therapy).

and hematological effects were managed effectively by dose reductions, growth factors, or transfusions. The largest study to date, from Oton and colleagues (65), treated 55 liver transplant recipients with recurrent HCV disease with peg-IFN-alpha-2b ($N = 51$) or peg-IFN-alpha-2a plus ribavirin for 48 weeks; they achieved EOTVR and SVR rates of 66.7% and 43.6%, respectively. Low baseline HCV-RNA ($p = 0.005$) and a length from transplantation to therapy between 2–4 years ($p = 0.011$) were predictors of SVR. Nonresponse was predicted by failure to achieve a viral load decrease at least $1 \log_{10}$ at week 4 and/or $2 \log_{10}$ at week 12. Toxicity led to treatment discontinuation in 16 patients (29%).

Tolerability of treatment remains a major limitation, even when used in stable patients several years from the time of transplantation. Dose reductions or drug discontinuation due to adverse effects are frequent. Maximum ribavirin doses achieved in studies to date are typically 200–600 mg lower than target doses used in nontransplant populations. Ribavirin pharmacokinetics are influenced by the frequent presence of renal impairment in liver transplant recipients. This is suggested by a study comparing ribavirin levels in 12 transplant recipients versus 15 nontransplant patients with chronic HCV on peg-IFN plus ribavirin (68). Baseline serum creatinine was higher: 1.27 versus 0.83 mg/dL in transplant compared to nontransplant patients. The ribavirin dose was lower in the transplant versus nontransplant patients (8.79 vs. 12.98 mg/kg/day), but plasma levels were the same in both groups (2.23 vs. 2.43 mg/L). Monitoring of ribavirin levels may facilitate more optimal dosing of ribavirin in liver transplant recipients, but such assays are not readily available. Thus, dosing of ribavirin in clinical practice is typically to the maximum dose tolerated with concurrent use of epoetin or darbopoetin alpha.

There is a theoretical risk of triggering acute rejection with the use of interferon. In uncontrolled trials of IFN and RBV combination therapy, the rate of acute rejection varies from 0% to 35% and the rate of chronic rejection varies from 0% to 4% (69). Controlled trials have shown no differences in rejection rates, but these studies were of limited sample size and small differences in rejection rates may be missed. Minimizing dose reductions of immunosuppressive agents during antiviral therapy and monitoring immunosuppressive drug levels and adjusting doses to maintain stable levels are potential means of minimizing the risk of intercurrent acute or chronic rejection.

In summary, peg-IFN plus ribavirin is the preferred treatment for recurrent HCV posttransplantation. Factors predictive of response include low baseline HCV RNA levels and early decline of HCV

RNA levels during treatment. Tolerability of therapy is limited, with discontinuations of 20% or higher. Measures to improve tolerability include the use of growth factors (epotein and filgrastim) and applying treatment in stable patients. Given the frequent complications of anemia and leukopenia during anti-HCV treatment, growth factors are usually needed. However, controlled studies establishing the benefits of adjuvant growth factor use in achieving improved tolerability, fewer dose reductions, or improved SVR rates are lacking. New therapies, which are more uniformly effective and better tolerated, are needed to improve rates of virologic response and ultimately reduce the rates of cirrhosis and graft loss.

SUMMARY

Recurrent infection is universal among transplant recipients who are viremic prior to transplantation, and the progression of histological disease is more rapid in the posttransplant setting. Factors contributing to accelerated disease progression are partially known, but many of these factors are not modifiable (e.g., donor age). The main therapeutic strategy for patients with recurrent HCV infection has been treatment with pegylated interferon and ribavirin once histological disease is evident. Overall response rates are lower than in nontransplant patients and treatment is less well tolerated. Peg-IFN combined with ribavirin is the treatment of choice. Preemptive antiviral therapy, initiated early after transplantation and prior to histological evidence of disease, offers no apparent advantage over treatment delayed until histological disease is present. Pretransplant antiviral therapy may be an option for selected patients with mildly decompensated cirrhosis. Achievement of an SVR prior to transplant prevents recurrence posttransplantation. Since treatment efficacy is lower and tolerability is limited in patients with decompensated cirrhosis, careful weighing of the risks versus benefits is needed and treatment only undertaken in an experienced transplant center. The need for new therapies for HCV-infected transplant recipients and patients with decompensated cirrhosis is urgent.

REFERENCES

1. Forman LM, Lewis JD, Berlin JA, Feldman HI, Lucey MR. The association between hepatitis C infection and survival after orthotopic liver transplantation. *Gastroenterology* 2002; 122(4):889–96.
2. Neumann UP, Berg T, Bahra M, Puhl G, Guckelberger O, Langrehr JM, et al. Long-term outcome of liver transplants for chronic hepatitis C: A 10-year follow-up. *Transplantation* 2004; 77(2):226–31.

3. Everhart J, Wei Y, Eng H, Charlton M, Persing D, Wiesner R, et al. Recurrent and new hepatitis C virus infection after liver transplantation. *Hepatology* 1999; 29:1220–6.

4. Prieto M, Berenguer M, Rayon J, Cordoba J, Arguello L, Carrasco D, et al. High incidence of allograft cirrhosis in hepatitis C virus genotype 1b infection following transplantation: Relationship with rejection episodes. *Hepatology* 1999; 29:250–6.

5. Gane E, Portmann B, Naoumov N, Smith H, Underhill J, Donaldson P, et al. Long-term outcome of hepatitis C infection after liver transplantation. *N Engl J Med* 1996; 334:815–20.

6. Feray C, Caccamo L, Alexander GJ, Ducot B, Gugenheim J, Casanovas T, et al. European collaborative study on factors influencing outcome after liver transplantation for hepatitis C. European Concerted Action on Viral Hepatitis (EUROHEP) Group. *Gastroenterology* 1999; 117(3):619–25.

7. Neumann U, Berg T, Bahra M, Seehofer D, Langrehr J, Neuhaus R, et al. Fibrosis progression after liver transplantation in patients with recurrent hepatitis C. *J Hepatol* 2004; 41(5):830–6.

8. Wali M, Harrison RF, Gow PJ, Mutimer D. Advancing donor liver age and rapid fibrosis progression following transplantation for hepatitis C. *Gut* 2002; 51(2): 248–52.

9. Berenguer M, Prieto M, Rayon JM, Mora J, Pastor M, Ortiz V, et al. Natural history of clinically compensated hepatitis C virus-related graft cirrhosis after liver transplantation. *Hepatology* 2000; 32(4 Pt 1):852–8.

10. Schluger L, Sheiner P, Thung S, Lau J, Min A, Wolf D, et al. Severe recurrent cholestatic hepatitis C following orthotopic liver transplantation. *Hepatology* 1996; 23:971–6.

11. Gaglio P, Malireddy S, Levitt B, Lapointe-Rudow D, Lefkowitch J, Kinkhabwala M, et al. Increased risk of cholestatic hepatitis C in recipients of grafts from living versus cadaveric liver donors. *Liver Transpl* 2003; 9(10): 1028–35.

12. Wali MH, Heydtmann M, Harrison RF, Gunson BK, Mutimer DJ. Outcome of liver transplantation for patients infected by hepatitis C, including those infected by genotype 4. *Liver Transpl* 2003; 9(8):796–804.

13. Berenguer M, Ferrell L, Watson J, Prieto M, Kim M, Rayon M, et al. HCV-related fibrosis progression following liver transplantation: Increase in recent years. *J Hepatol* 2000; 32(4):673–84.

14. Burak KW, Kremers WK, Batts KP, Wiesner RH, Rosen CB, Razonable RR, et al. Impact of cytomegalovirus infection, year of transplantation, and donor age on outcomes after liver transplantation for hepatitis C. *Liver Transpl* 2002; 8(4): 362–9.

15. Lake JR, Shorr JS, Steffen BJ, Chu AH, Gordon RD, Wiesner RH. Differential effects of donor age in liver transplant recipients infected with hepatitis B, hepatitis C and without viral hepatitis. *Am J Transpl* 2005; 5(3):549–57.

16. Sheiner P, Schwartz M, Mor E, Schluger L, Theise N, Kishikawa K, et al. Severe and multiple rejection episodes are associated with early recurrence of hepatitis C after orthotopic liver transplantation. *Hepatology* 1995; 21(1):30–4.

17. Rosen HR, Chou S, Corless CL, Gretch DR, Flora KD, Boudousquie A, et al. Cytomegalovirus viremia: Risk factor for allograft cirrhosis after liver transplantation for hepatitis C. *Transplantation* 1997; 64(5):721–6.

18. Charlton M, Seaberg E, Wiesner R, Everhart J, Zetterman R, Lake J, et al. Predictors of patient and graft survival following liver transplantation for hepatitis C. *Hepatology* 1998; 28:823–30.

19. Wiesner R, Sorrell M, Villamil F, International Liver Transplantation Society Expert Panel. Report of the First International Liver Transplantation Society Expert Panel Consensus Conference on liver transplantation and hepatitis C. *Liver Transpl* 2003; 9(11):S1–S9.

20. Terrault NA, Berenguer M. Treating hepatitis C infection in liver transplant recipients. *Liver Transpl* 2006; 12(8):1192–204.

21. Terrault NA, Shiffman ML, Lok AS, et al. Outcomes in hepatitis C virus-infected recipients of living donor vs. deceased donor liver transplantation. *Liver Transpl* 2007; 13(1):122–9.

22. Garcia-Retortillo M, Forns X, Llovet J, Navasa M, Feliu A, Massaguer A, et al. Hepatitis C recurrence is more severe after living donor compared to cadaveric liver transplantation. *Hepatology* 2004; 40(3):699–707.

23. Shiffman M, Stravitz R, Contos M, Mills A, Sterling R, Luketic V, et al. Histologic recurrence of chronic hepatitis C virus in patients after living donor and deceased donor liver transplantation. *Liver Transpl* 2004; 10:1248–55.

24. Watashi K, Hijikata M, Hosaka M, Yamaji M, Shimotohno K. Cyclosporin A suppresses replication of hepatitis C virus genome in cultured hepatocytes. *Hepatology* 2003; 38(5):1282–8.

25. Levy G, Villamil F, Samuel D, Sanjuan F, Grazi GL, Wu Y, et al. Results of LIS2T, a multicenter, randomized study comparing cyclosporine microemulsion with C2 monitoring and tacrolimus with C0 monitoring in de novo liver transplantation. *Transplantation* 2004; 77(11):1632–8.

26. Martin P, Busuttil RW, Goldstein RM, Crippin JS, Klintmalm GB, Fitzsimmons WE, et al. Impact of tacrolimus versus cyclosporine in hepatitis C virus-infected liver transplant recipients on recurrent hepatitis: A prospective, randomized trial. *Liver Transpl* 2004; 10(10):1258–62.

27. Fisher RA, Stone JJ, Wolfe LG, Rodgers CM, Anderson ML, Sterling RK, et al. Four-year follow-up of a prospective randomized trial of mycophenolate mofetil with cyclosporine microemulsion or tacrolimus following liver transplantation. *Clin Transpl* 2004; 18(4):463–72.

28. Berenguer M, Aguilera V, Prieto M, San Juan F, Rayon JM, Benlloch S, et al. Significant improvement in the outcome of HCV-infected transplant recipients by avoiding rapid steroid tapering and potent induction immunosuppression. *J Hepatol* 2006; 44(4):717–22.

29. Hilgard P, Kahraman A, Lehmann N, Seltmann C, Beckebaum S, Ross RS, et al. Cyclosporine versus tacrolimus in patients with HCV infection after liver transplantation: Effects on virus replication and recurrent hepatitis. *World J Gastroenterol* 2006; 12(5):697–702.

30. Bahra M, Neumann UI, Jacob D, Puhl G, Klupp J, Langrehr JM, et al. MMF and calcineurin taper in recurrent hepatitis C after liver transplantation: Impact on histological course. *Am J Transpl* 2005; 5(2):406–11.

31. Zekry A, Gleeson M, Guney S, McCaughan GW. A prospective cross-over study comparing the effect of mycophenolate versus azathioprine on allograft function and viral load in liver transplant recipients with recurrent chronic HCV infection. *Liver Transpl* 2004; 10(1):52–7.

32. Wiesner RH, Shorr JS, Steffen BJ, Chu AH, Gordon RD, Lake JR. Mycophenolate mofetil combination therapy improves long-term outcomes after liver transplantation in patients with and without hepatitis C. *Liver Transpl* 2005; 11(7):750–9.

33. Filipponi F, Callea F, Salizzoni M, Grazi GL, Fassati LR, Rossi M, et al. Double-blind comparison of hepatitis C histological recurrence rate in HCV+ liver transplant recipients given basiliximab + steroids or basiliximab + placebo, in addition to cyclosporine and azathioprine. *Transplantation* 2004; 78(10):1488–95.

34. Eason JD, Nair S, Cohen AJ, Blazek JL, Loss GE, Jr. Steroid-free liver transplantation using rabbit antithymocyte globulin and early tacrolimus monotherapy. *Transplantation* 2003; 75(8):1396–9.

35. Brillanti S, Vivarelli M, De Ruvo N, Aden AA, Camaggi V, D'Errico A, et al. Slowly tapering off steroids protects the graft against hepatitis C recurrence after liver transplantation. *Liver Transpl* 2002; 8(10):884–8.

36. Belli L, Alberti A, Vangeli M, Airoldi A, Pinzello G. Tapering off steroids three months after liver transplantation is not detrimental for hepatitis C virus disease recurrence. *Liver Transpl* 2003; 9(2):201–2.

37. Papatheodoridis GV, Davies S, Dhillon AP, Teixeira R, Goulis J, Davidson B, et al. The role of different immunosuppression in the long-term histological outcome of HCV reinfection after liver transplantation for HCV cirrhosis. *Transplantation* 2001; 72(3):412–8.

38. Gonzalez MG, Madrazo CP, Rodriguez AB, Gutierrez MG, Herrero JI, Pallardo JM, et al. An open, randomized, multicenter clinical trial of oral tacrolimus in liver allograft transplantation: A comparison of dual vs. triple drug therapy. *Liver Transpl* 2005; 11(5):515–24.

39. Tisone G, Orlando G, Cardillo A, Palmieri G, Manzia TM, Baiocchi L, et al. Complete weaning off immunosuppression in HCV liver transplant recipients is feasible and favourably impacts on the progression of disease recurrence. *J Hepatol* 2006; 44:702–9.

40. Everson G. Treatment of patients with hepatitis C virus on the waiting list. *Hepatology* 2005; in press.

41. Forns X, Navasa M, Rodes J. Treatment of HCV infection in patients with advanced cirrhosis. *Hepatology* 2004; 40(2):498.

42. Davis G, Nelson D, Terrault N, Pruett T, Schiano T, Fletcher C, et al. A randomized, open-label study to evaluate the safety and pharmacokinetics of human hepatitis C immune globulin (Civacir) in liver transplant recipients. *Liver Transpl* 2005; in press.

43. Schiano TD, Charlton M, Younassi Z, et al. A phase III study of monoclonal antibody HCV-ABXTL-68 in patients requiring liver transplant for HCV disease. *Hepatology* 2005; 42:A701.

44. Khalili M, Vardanian AJ, Hamerski CM, Wang R, Bacchetti P, Roberts JP, et al. Management of hepatitis C-infected liver transplant recipients at large North American centres: Changes in recent years. *Clin Transpl* 2006; 20(1):1–9.

45. Regev A, Molina E, Moura R, Bejarano PA, Khaled A, Ruiz P, et al. Reliability of histopathologic assessment for the differentiation of recurrent hepatitis C from acute rejection after liver transplantation. *Liver Transpl* 2004; 10(10):1233–9.

46. Netto GJ, Watkins DL, Williams JW, Colby TV, dePetris G, Sharkey FE, et al. Interobserver agreement in hepatitis C grading and staging and in the Banff grading schema for acute cellular rejection: The "Hepatitis C 3" Multi-Institutional Trial experience. *Arch Pathol Lab Med* 2006; 130(8):1157–62.

47. Crippin JS, McCashland T, Terrault N, Sheiner P, Charlton MR. A pilot study of the tolerability and efficacy of antiviral therapy in hepatitis C virus-infected patients awaiting liver transplantation. *Liver Transpl* 2002; 8(4):350–5.

48. Singh N, Gayowski T, Wannstedt CF, Shakil AO, Wagener MM, Fung JJ, et al. Interferon-alpha for prophylaxis of recurrent viral hepatitis C in liver transplant recipients: A prospective, randomized, controlled trial. *Transplantation* 1998; 65(1):82–6.

49. Sheiner P, Boros P, Klion F, Thung S, Schluger L, Lau J, et al. The efficacy of prophylactic interferon alfa-2b in preventing recurrent hepatitis C after liver transplantation. *Hepatology* 1998; 28:831–8.

50. Chalasani N, Manzarbeitia C, Ferenci P, Vogel W, Fontana RJ, Voigt M, et al. Peginterferon alfa-2a for hepatitis C after liver transplantation: Two randomized, controlled trials. *Hepatology* 2005; 41(2):289–98.

51. Shergill A, Khalili M, Straley S, Bollinger K, Roberts J, Ascher N, et al. Applicability, tolerability and efficacy of preemptive antiviral therapy in hepatitis C infected patients undergoing liver transplantation. *Am J Transpl* 2005; 5(1): 118–24.

52. Sugawara Y, Makuuchi M, Matsui Y, Kishi Y, Akamatsu N, Kaneko J, et al. Preemptive therapy for hepatitis C virus after living-donor liver transplantation. *Transplantation* 2004; 78(9):1308–11.

53. Mazzaferro V, Tagger A, Schiavo M, Regalia E, Pulvirenti A, Ribero ML, et al. Prevention of recurrent hepatitis C after liver transplantation with early interferon and ribavirin treatment. *Transpl Proc* 2001; 33(1–2):1355–7.

54. Terrault NA. Treatment of recurrent hepatitis C in liver transplant recipients. *Clin Gastroenterol Hepatol* 2005; 3(10 Suppl 2):S125–S131.

55. Gane E, Lo S, Portmann B, Lau J, Naoumov N, Williams R. A randomized study of the safety and efficacy of ribavirin versus interferon monotherapy for recurrent HCV infection in liver transplant recipients. *Hepatology* 1998; 24(4 Pt 2):293A.

56. Wright T, Combs C, Kim M, Ferrell L, Bacchetti P, Ascher N, et al. Interferon-alpha therapy for hepatitis C virus infection after liver transplantation. *Hepatology* 1994; 20(4):773–9.

57. Giostra E, Kullak-Ublick G, Keller W, Fried R, Vanlemmens C, Kraehenbuhl S, et al. Ribavirin/interferon-alpha sequential treatment of recurrent hepatitis C after liver transplantation. *Transpl Int* 2004; 17(4):169–76.

58. Firpi R, Abdelmalek M, Soldevila-Pico C, Reed A, Hemming A, Howard R, et al. Combination of interferon alfa-2b and ribavirin in liver transplant recipients with histological recurrent hepatitis C. *Liver Transpl* 2002; 8(11):1000–6.

59. Mukherjee S, Lyden E, McCashland TM, Schafer DF. Interferon alpha 2b and ribavirin for the treatment of recurrent hepatitis C after liver transplantation: Cohort study of 38 patients. *J Gastroenterol Hepatol* 2005; 20(2):198–203.

60. Samuel D, Bizollon T, Feray C, Roche B, Ahmed S, Lemonnier C, et al. Interferon-alpha 2b plus ribavirin in patients with chronic hepatitis C after liver transplantation: A randomized study. *Gastroenterology* 2003; 124(3):642–50.

61. Bizollon T, Ahmed S, Radenne S, Chevallier M, Chevallier P, Parvaz P, et al. Long term histological improvement and clearance of intrahepatic hepatitis C virus RNA following sustained response to interferon-ribavirin combination therapy in liver transplanted patients with hepatitis C virus recurrence. *Gut* 2003; 52:283–7.

62. Dumortier J, Scoazec J, Chevallier P, Boillot O. Treatment of recurrent hepatitis C after liver transplantation: A pilot study of peginterferon alfa-2b and ribavirin combination. *J Hepatol* 2004; 40(4):669–74.

63. Abdelmalek M, Firpi R, Soldevila-Pico C, Reed A, Hemming A, Liu C, et al. Sustained viral response to interferon and ribavirin in liver transplant recipients with recurrent hepatitis C. *Liver Transpl* 2004; 10(2):199–207.

64. Berenguer M, Prieto M, Palau A, Carrasco D, Rayon JM, Calvo F, et al. Recurrent hepatitis C genotype 1b following liver transplantation: Treatment with combination interferon-ribavirin therapy. *Eur J Gastroenterol Hepatol* 2004; 16(11): 1207–12.

65. Oton E, Barcena R, Moreno-Planas JM, Cuervas-Mons V, Moreno-Zamora A, Barrios C, et al. Hepatitis C recurrence after liver transplantation: Viral and histologic response to full-dose peg-interferon and ribavirin. *Am J Transpl* 2006; 6:2348–55.

66. Castells L, Vargas V, Allende H, Bilbao I, Luis Lázaro J, Margarit C, et al. Combined treatment with pegylated interferon (alpha-2b) and ribavirin in the acute phase of hepatitis C virus recurrence after liver transplantation. *J Hepatol* 2005; 43:53–9.

67. Rodriguez-Luna H, Khatib A, Sharma P, De Petris G, Williams JW, Ortiz J, et al. Treatment of recurrent hepatitis C infection after liver transplantation with combination of pegylated interferon alpha2b and ribavirin: An open-label series. *Transplantation* 2004; 77(2):190–4.

68. Dumortier J, Ducos E, Scoazec JY, Chevallier P, Boillot O, Gagnieu MC. Plasma ribavirin concentrations during treatment of recurrent hepatitis C with peginterferon alpha-2b and ribavirin combination after liver transplantation. *J Viral Hepat* 2006; 13(8):538–43.

69. Biggins SW, Terrault NA. Treatment of recurrent hepatitis C after liver transplantation. *Clin Liver Dis* 2005; 9(3):505–23, ix.

4 The Dilemma of Adult-to-Adult Living Donor Liver Transplantation

John F. Renz, MD, PhD
and Robert S. Brown Jr., MD, MPH

CONTENTS

INTRODUCTION
HISTORICAL BACKGROUND
DONOR OUTCOMES
RECIPIENT OUTCOMES
DISCUSSION
REFERENCES

Abstract

Adult-to-adult living donor liver transplantation (aLDLT) has rapidly evolved in less than a decade. In countries with a robust deceased donor-organ allocation, only about 3–4% of all liver transplantations are aLDLT. Several types of living donor grafts may be utilized for aLDLT. The donor morbidity and mortality represent short- and long-term impediments to further application of aLDLT, and our understanding of the donor risks associated with this procedure continues to evolve. The outcomes of aLDLT are favorable, and pursuing aLDLT may offer a survival *advantage* compared to candidates who do not have a potential living donor. The application

From: *Clinical Gastroenterology: Liver Transplantation: Challenging Controversies and Topics*
Edited by: G. T. Everson and J. F. Trotter, DOI: 10.1007/978-1-60327-028-1_4,
© Humana Press, Totowa, NJ

of aLDLT in different regions of the world is discussed. In addition, the special issues related to aLDLT in patients with hepatocellular carcinoma and those infected with hepatitis C are reviewed.

Key Words: Living donor liver transplantation; Donor complications; Hepatocellular carcinoma; Liver allocation

INTRODUCTION

Adult-to-adult living donor liver transplantation (aLDLT) is a remarkable technical achievement designed to increase organ supply. Justification of living donation originates from increasing waitlist morbidity and mortality among transplant candidates (1). With over 800 European, 1,600 North American, and 2,000 Asian aLDLT procedures reported, living donor liver transplantation for adults has been performed and reported throughout the world (2, 3). The rapid evolution of these surgical strategies has occurred in less than a decade and has spawned new areas of discovery that impact liver transplantation as well as hepatobiliary surgery (4, 5). This includes the medical management of recipients with "small-for-size" allografts (6, 7), the treatment of complications unique to partial-allograft transplantation (5, 8–12), liver regeneration in donors and recipients (13, 14), and postdonation donor management (15–21).

Application of aLDLT in countries with a robust deceased donor-organ allocation scheme has reached a plateau at approximately 3–4% of all transplant procedures performed (3, 22). Barriers to increases in living donation to the level seen in kidney transplantation (~50% of all transplant procedures performed) are numerous and varied, as detailed below. Sustained application of aLDLT has unfortunately yielded inevitable donor morbidity and mortality that continues to stimulate ethical debate as to the future of these procedures (23, 24). Following a brief review of the historical background of aLDLT, this chapter summarizes current aLDLT outcomes through May 2006 and postulates evidence-based strategies to optimize its utilization.

HISTORICAL BACKGROUND

Liver transplantation utilizing a partial-liver allograft was theoretically proposed for children by Smith in 1969 (25) and first successfully performed by Raia in 1989 (26). LDLT in children originated as a response to the disparity in pediatric waitlist times that resulted in pediatric waitlist mortality exceeding 25% (27, 28). Strong was the first to perform pediatric living donor liver transplantation (pLDLT) with long-term success (29) and Broelsch reported the first clinical series of pLDLT (30). Through the 1990s, pLDLT was broadly applied throughout the world with results that equaled or exceeded deceased whole-allograft transplantation in infants. Surgical techniques acquired through pLDLT were later introduced to deceased donation to create split-liver transplantation: the creation of an adult and pediatric allograft from a single deceased donor (31).

Application of pLDLT significantly increased organ availability, lowered waitlist morbidity, and fundamentally changed medical practice with respect to the transplantation of children. Transplantation of children could occur as an *elective* procedure and could be timed to minimize the impact of liver disease upon a child's growth and development. Accordingly, pLDLT has enjoyed continued growth and evolution to become the preferred allograft for children less than 3 years of age (32, 33).

The success of pLDLT, coupled with exponential increasing demand among potential adult transplant recipients during the late 1990s leading to ever-rising waiting times and as a result waitlist morbidity and mortality, provided a powerful stimulus to extend the use of living donation to adult recipients (34, 35). However, the application of living donor liver transplantation to adults mandates unique surgical and medical considerations. The principal surgical challenges include the procurement of an allograft with sufficient liver volume to meet the metabolic needs of the recipient, positioning of the allograft to optimize vascular inflow, venous outflow, and biliary drainage, as well as an appreciation of anatomical variations that necessitate complex biliary or vascular reconstruction (15).

Several allografts are available for aLDLT; the specific choice of allograft is significant as each predisposes the recipient and donor to a unique set of potential complications. Potential complications that require special attention include biliary complications, bleeding of the cut-liver surface, acute and chronic hepatic venous outflow obstruction, hepatic arterial complications, and poor synthetic function secondary to insufficient hepatic residual volume in the donor or insufficient transplanted allograft volume to fulfill the recipient's metabolic demands.

The anatomical classification of the liver described by Couinaud (36) and refined by Bismuth (37) has been universally accepted by the transplant communities of Europe, Asia, and North America as the reference system for describing allografts created by LDLT. The four anatomical allografts utilized for LDLT (Fig. 1) include the entire right liver lobe (Couinaud segments V–VIII), the entire left liver lobe (Couinaud

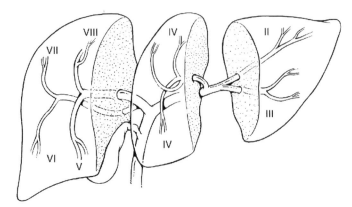

Fig. 1. Surgical division of the liver yields a left lobe (segments I–IV) and a right (segments V–VIII) lobe, which can be utilized in split- and adult-to-adult living-donor liver transplantation. Alternate division along the falciform ligament yields the pediatric left lateral segment allograft (segments II and III) and the adult extended right lobe allograft (segments IV–VIII).

segments II–IV), the left lateral segment (Couinaud segments II and III), and the extended right liver or "trisegment" allograft (Couinaud segments IV–VIII).

While all four allografts have been successfully applied to select adult recipients (38, 39), the right lobe allograft, accounting for greater than 60% of the donor's total liver mass, is the most commonly employed allograft for aLDLT worldwide and will be the default allograft for the remainder of this chapter unless otherwise specified. Right lobe allografts generally permit equal-sized donor-to-recipient weight ratios or even slightly smaller donors to donate to larger recipients. Utilization of a right lobe allograft was initially described by Habib and Tanaka of Kyoto, who were attempting to harvest a left lobe for LDLT when anatomical considerations favored a right lobe hepatectomy (40). Wachs of the University of Colorado was the first to describe LDLT utilizing a right lobe allograft in North America (41).

The left lobe allograft (Couinaud segments II–IV) accounts for approximately 35% of total liver volume and typically provides 300–500-cc allografts. These allografts are commonly utilized for smaller adults or older adolescents with recipient weights of approximately 50 kg.

Transplantation of the left lateral segment (Couinaud segments II and III) to select larger children and adult recipients has been performed in the setting of large donor-to-recipient size disparity. The volume of the left lateral segment typically accounts for approximately 20% of the standard liver volume and yields a 200–300-cc allograft. In the authors' experience, the upper limit of recipient weight for living donation of left lateral segment allografts has been less than 40 kg. These parameters clearly limit the applicability of left lateral segment allografts to a small subgroup of adult recipients.

The least commonly applied aLDLT allograft is the extended right lobe derived from Couinaud segments IV–VIII (42, 43). Extended right lobe allografts account for greater than 70% of the standard liver volume and permit relatively small donors to donate to larger recipients. Retrospective analysis of donor risks comparing extended right lobectomy versus left lobectomy found extended right procedures resulted in significantly increased donor liver dysfunction with prolonged cholestasis and the development of biliary strictures (43). In the opinion of most experts, while extended right donor lobectomy has been refined to reduce the incidence of donor complications (44), the potential risks to the donor of removing over three fourths of his or her liver cannot currently justify widespread utilization of this technique.

Medical and surgical considerations include the management of biliary complications, complications from bleeding of the cut-liver surface, acute and chronic hepatic venous outflow obstruction, hepatic arterial complications, and poor allograft function secondary to insufficient hepatic volume to meet immediate metabolic needs, termed "small-for-size syndrome."

"Small-for-size syndrome" is characterized by synthetic dysfunction, increased serum transaminases typically two to four times the upper limit of normal, and prolonged cholestasis frequently accompanied by continued ascites production (6). The time course for improved synthetic function typically occurs within 72 hours of transplantation, as the allograft undergoes rapid hypertrophy, while cholestasis typically improves over the course of weeks to months. In the recipient, the occurrence of only these symptoms without the need for augmentation of synthetic function predicts a reversible situation that will improve as the allograft undergoes regeneration; however, the appearance of encephalopathy, hypoglycemia, or metabolic acidosis or the continued need for augmentation of synthetic function beyond 48 hours heralds irreversible allograft failure that should prompt evaluation for retransplantation.

Small-for-size syndrome in a donor requires immediate and careful assessment. Clinical management during the precarious period of hepatic regeneration should be directed at minimizing additional metabolic demand secondary to infection, unnecessary surgery, or iatrogenic injury while optimizing donor physiology with respect to tissue perfusion, coagulation, vasopressor utilization, acid-base balance, fluids, and electrolyte repletion (23, 24, 45). When a donor is experiencing limited metabolic reserve, the a priori assignment of specific criteria for response, such as requirement for intubation or need for augmented synthetic function beyond 48 hours resulting in listing for liver transplantation, serves to guide clinical management and alleviate uncertainty among the staff and donor's family. Listing a donor for possible liver transplantation is a very serious commitment; however, if necessary, early transplantation in the setting of hepatic insufficiency may avoid the mortality from multisystem organ failure that can result from the natural path of human indecision when faced with such a calamity.

Biopsy of small-for-size allografts reveals a characteristic pattern of diffuse ischemic injury demonstrated by hepatocyte ballooning, steatosis, centrilobular necrosis, and parenchymal cholestasis that is frequently misinterpreted as preservation injury (6). As the allograft recovers, normalization of biopsy specimens typically occurs within two weeks of transplantation, except for the presence of cholestasis, which typically persists for longer than one month. While radiologic data from Kawasaki (13) and Nakagami (14) demonstrate the majority of volume regeneration occurring within seven days of living donor liver transplantation, the small-for-size allograft should be considered highly vulnerable to insult, with an increased risk of developing significant sequelae from complications or additional metabolic stress in the immediate postoperative period. Pomfret has reported the most sophisticated analysis of donor and recipient regenerative patterns for aLDLT that evolve for up to one year following surgery (46). Portal hypertensive physiology and clinical cholestasis will typically resolve over a period of several weeks.

No formal registry for long-term or detailed short-term follow-up on aLDLT has been successfully implemented despite widespread calls for its creation (47–51). The National Institutes of Health (NIH) has supported a multicenter study on aLDLT (A2ALL) (52). To date, the nine-center group has reported some retrospective multicenter data; however, prospective data collection is still at an early stage. Thus, detailed data on the performance of aLDLT exist only as individual reports in the literature.

DONOR OUTCOMES

ALDLT is practiced throughout the world, including in Asia, North America, South America, Europe, and the Middle East. Presently, the reported worldwide incidence of right lobe aLDLT exceeds 3,000. With this experience, aLDLT donor outcome data are slowly emerging. As expected, the incidence and severity of aLDLT donor complications are higher than those reported for pediatric donation (49) because of the significantly more difficult surgical procedure performed upon a wider spectrum of donor candidates (23, 24, 45). Direct technical comparisons are invalid, as the procurement of a right lobe, extended right lobe, or left lobe is substantially more difficult than the procurement of a left lateral segment allograft. The donor undergoes a larger operation for a longer period of time and donates a much larger fraction of available hepatic parenchyma. The result is less metabolic reserve to maintain homeostasis or recover from a complication.

In addition, most pediatric donor candidates are parents, which narrows the population with respect to age and relationship. aLDLT includes a more heterogeneous population with variable age, health, physical, and emotional attachment to the potential recipient. Donor candidates may range from a teenage or adult child of the potential recipient to an older spouse, parent, sibling, or friend. Liver regeneration and postdonation physiological data derived from pLDLT are of limited applicability over such a diverse population.

The lack of a formal registry outside the undergoing A2ALL study impedes verifiable donor outcome data on aLDLT. Unfortunately, scarce data exist on long-term donor outcomes (53–56). A survey of U.S. transplant centers revealed widespread variation in practice patterns on long-term follow-up for aLDLT donors (54). During the first year, 68% exercised a formal follow-up protocol; however, greater than one-year follow-up was typically "as needed," with appointments initiated by the donor (57). While multiple reports indicate average hospital stays of less than seven days and the performance of living donation without the need for nonautologous blood transfusions, serious donor complications and death are possible (38, 41, 57). Complications related to anesthesia, performance of surgery, surgical technique, postoperative recovery, metabolic stress of liver regeneration, impaired wound healing, as well as the psychosocial impact of major surgery and recovery have become evident with the increasing clinical experience of aLDLT (58). Marcos and Todo each reported no significant donor complications in early series of 40 and 27 right lobe allografts, respectively (59, 60), while Testa reported an overall complication rate of greater than 50% in the performance of 30 right lobe allografts (61). An ASTS survey of 30 North American transplant centers that performed 208 aLDLT in 2000 identified an overall donor complication rate of 10% (23). The most common donor complication was hernia and wound infection, with a less than

Table 1
Donor Complications of Pediatric Living Donor Liver Transplantation

Author	Year	N	Follow-up (yr)	Complication (%)
Lo (62)	2003	605	5	9
Grewal (21)	1998	100	3	34
Ohkohchi (19)	1998	25	3	40
Yamaoka (63)	1995	100	2	15
Malago (64)	1994	36	2	19

5% incidence of postoperative biliary leak that was typically treated by percutaneous drainage. Infrequent complications included pressure sores, pulmonary embolus, pneumonia, and symptomatic pleural effusion. Approximately 5% of donors require heterologous blood transfusion, and 3% of donors required reoperation for complications related to donation (23).

Many centers and surveys have subsequently reported similar donor complications, with a very wide incidence ranging from 18 to 40% (Table 1). Additional serious donor complications reported include portal vein thrombosis, neuropraxia, pleural effusion, ascites, pneumonia, and abortion of the living donor procedure because of intraoperative findings (2, 23, 24, 45). Existing data on donor complications are summarized in Table 2. The discrepancy observed in the incidence of donor complications demonstrates the inherent limitations of retrospective surveys and underscores the limitations of existing data in the absence of a verifiable data collection instrument.

A donor outcome survey from five Asian centers including 334 left lobe and 561 right lobe aLDLT was reported by Lo (62). Right lobe donors experienced a 28% overall complication rate that was higher than left lobe (7%) or left lateral segment (9%) allograft donors. Complications included cholestasis (7%), bile leak (6%), biliary stricture (1%), portal vein thrombosis (0.5%), intra-abdominal bleeding (0.5%), and pulmonary embolism (0.5%). There was no hospital mortality, but there was a late donor death three years after donation. Long-term follow-up information was only available from 15% of the donor population (62).

Extended right lobe donors experience more significant complications. In an early series, Lo reported a donor survival of 100%; however, significant donor complications were observed, including infection, prolonged cholestasis, bile leak, and late biliary stricture (43). Retrospective analysis of donor risks comparing extended right lobectomy versus left lobectomy found donors who had undergone an extended right procedure exhibited more significant transient liver dysfunction with two donors developing cholestasis due to biliary strictures. Although the technique has been refined to reduce the complication rate (44), the potential risks incurred to donors by removing over three fourths of their liver mandate limitation of this technique to highly select circumstances.

Donor death and emergent transplantation have been reported in North America, Europe, and Asia. Although the precise number of donor deaths to date is speculative (2, 24, 45, 65, 66), donor mortality is an expected occurrence in aLDLT. Based on existing data, a reasonable estimate of the incidence of donor mortality is 0.4% (1, 2, 23). This is fundamentally different from living donor kidney or left lateral segment donation, where donor mortality *must* be the result of a significant negative-impact event. In aLDLT, liver failure is an inherent component of the procedure because of the inability to predict hepatic regeneration a priori. Without the ability to predict hepatic regeneration, the donor operation is flawed. Therefore, the procedure can be performed with complete technical precision and without a negative-impact event, yet yield a negative outcome.

Donor morbidity and mortality represent short- and long-term impediments to further application of aLDLT. Performance of aLDLT exposes a liver transplant program to significant negative consequences that can affect deceased donor transplantation in the event of serious donor morbidity or mortality. As expected, donor mortality in the immediate postoperative period has stimulated institutional and governmental quality reviews, recommendations, and policy implementation. However,

Table 2
Complications of Adult-to-Adult Living Donor Transplantation Series Data

Complications	Incidence (%)
Overall	15–50
Biliary leak	8–15
Rehospitalization	~8
Small-for-size	~5
Reoperation	~5
Biliary stricture	~3
Bowel obstruction	~3
Pulmonary embolus	~2

long-term donor quality of life and outcomes represent an equally significant challenge that has yet to be appreciated. To date, no long-term donor outcome data exist from a study that ensures confidentiality. The subject has been evaluated with respect to living donor kidney donation and the results are likely transferable. In a seminal study by Simmons et al., the majority of kidney living donors reported enhanced self-esteem and a willingness to donate again (67). The same was true in a confidential study of pLDLT donors by Diaz et al. (68). However, long-term, large cohort studies among kidney living donors have identified predictors of donor dissatisfaction through multivariate analysis (69). Repeatedly, donors other than first-degree relatives and recipient death within one year following living donor kidney transplantation were associated with donor dissatisfaction (67, 69). Interestingly, parents who donated to their children consistently demonstrated the highest level of satisfaction, a finding mirrored in pLDLT donor literature (68). Parent-to-child donation is a minority of aLDLT. The wide range of relationships between aLDLT donors and recipients, combined with other first-degree relationships among donors such as spouse or children who receive less direct benefit from the act of donation, introduces significant potential for overall dissatisfaction with the process in the event of a complication.

Precise morbidity and mortality data along with detailed donor satisfaction outcomes are addressed in detail by the A2ALL study and have been incorporated in the development of Japanese and European registries; however, prospective data have not matured. These data are essential to accurately assess and weigh donor risk versus substantial benefit through decreased morbidity and improved overall mortality for candidates with a potential donor (70).

RECIPIENT OUTCOMES

Left Lobe Allografts

Makuuchi et al. were the first to report successful aLDLT utilizing a left lobe allograft (38), with the largest North American series reported by Miller of Mt. Sinai Medical Center, New York (39). While complications and allograft survival among left lobe recipients have paralleled those of right lobe recipients, transplantation of left lobe allografts is technically more difficult than right lobe allografts. Technical challenges of left lobe allografts include greater anatomical variance, smaller transplanted volumes, and increased difficulty in precise anatomical allograft positioning as a result of the left-to-right orientation of hilar structures.

North American and European Outcomes

The Annual Report of the U.S. Scientific Registry of Transplant Recipients (SRTR) and the Organ Procurement and Transplant Network identifies 253 aLDLT performed among 5,125 total liver transplants in 2005 (71). aLDLT peaked at 408 procedures in 2001 (71). SRTR data are limited to the performance of a procedure and previously did not identify the type of allograft utilized or detail outcomes; however, the right lobe allograft (Couinaud segments V–VIII) is utilized in the majority of procedures. In North America, the average adult body habitus excludes utilization of left lobe allografts that are typically restricted to a recipient body mass of less than 60 kg. Wachs of the University of Colorado was the first to describe aLDLT utilizing a right lobe allograft in North America (41). In an initial series of 40 right lobe allografts, Marcos et al. reported an 80% recipient survival in their first 20 recipients that improved to 95% during the performance of the second group of 20 recipients (59). Bak of the University of Colorado reported an 85% recipient survival in an initial series of 20 right lobe allografts (72). Multiple detailed reviews have followed (3, 45, 73, 74). Individual center reports from the literature are summarized in Table 3.

The American Society of Transplant Surgeons initiated the earliest attempt to create a registry identifying outcomes of aLDLT within North America. A data-protected survey was distributed to all transplant centers within the United States and Canada that contribute to the UNOS database. The overall response exceeded 88% and identified 30 North

Table 3
Living Donor Liver Transplantation in the United States; Right Lobe Allografts

Center	Author	Year	N	Recip	Graft	Comp
New York (75)	Miller	2003	99	92%	88%	38%
Los Angeles (76)	Ghobrial	2002	20	95%	85%	39%
New York (77)	Fishbein	2001	50	87%	80%	32%
Denver (72)	Bak	2001	41	93%	88%	>34%
New York (78)	Goldstein	2001	20	75%	55%	30%
Chapel Hill (79)	Fair	2001	14	93%	78%	N/A
Memphis (80)	Grewal	2001	11	91%	88%	63%
Rochester (59)	Marcos	2000	40	88%	85%	47%
Richmond (81)	Marcos	1999	25	88%	88%	52%

Recip = recipient one-year survival; Graft = graft one-year survival; Comp = incidence of complications.

American liver transplant centers that had performed a total of 208 aLDLT (1). Twenty-eight (13%) aLDLT recipient deaths were reported: Fourteen (6%) were related to allograft dysfunction, 10 (5%) were unrelated to allograft function, and 4 (2%) were undetermined. Recipient deaths not attributed to allograft function included intracranial hemorrhage, myocardial infarction, hemolytic-uremic syndrome, recurrent hepatitis C, graft-versus-host disease, multiple myeloma, recurrent hepatoma, recidivism, and *aspergillosis* six months following aLDLT.

Sixty-three complications were reported, yielding an overall complication incidence of 30% (1). The three most frequent complications reported were biliary, vascular, and primary allograft nonfunction. Thirty-seven biliary complications were reported (for an incidence of 18%), including parenchymal bile leak, biliary anastomotic leak, and biliary anastomotic strictures. Vascular complications resulted in the loss of four allografts, with an overall 6% incidence of complications including aneurysm, anastomotic stricture, and hepatic arterial thrombosis. Ten allografts (4%) were lost to primary nonfunction. Additional surgical complications included two Roux-limb leaks and one duodenal ulcer requiring surgery. The incidence of complications did not correlate with the annual number of deceased donor whole-organ transplants performed by an individual center but did improve among centers with a greater experience of aLDLT, reflecting the "learning-curve" effect (44, 59, 72, 82). The overall incidence of allograft failure was 12%, including primary nonfunction and recipient deaths due to allograft failure or complications. These data are in agreement with the 10% incidence of allograft failure reported by Broelsch (83) and notably better than the 19% incidence of allograft loss reported by Inomata (84).

Brown conducted a later survey of U.S. transplant programs and reported data on 449 aLDLT (85). Centers that performed aLDLT were more likely to have larger deceased donor volumes and experience in pediatric transplantation. Although recipient and allograft survival were not reported, the reported incidence of biliary and vascular complications was 23% and 8%, respectively.

Fishbein performed an analysis of the impact of aLDLT upon transplant volume and demographics in UNOS Region 9 (New York) (77). The State of New York shares a single waiting list but has five programs offering aLDLT. During the period from August 1998 through November 2000, the volume of deceased donor allografts was unchanged, while the proportion of living donor allografts increased from 2.2% of total transplants performed to 28%, yielding a net increase of 118 allografts (77). The overall actuarial one-year recipient and allograft survival were 84% and 78%, respectively, demonstrating a learning-curve effect. Notably, the incidence of emergent retransplantation as a UNOS status 1 for allograft primary nonfunction was 7.8% for aLDLT allografts versus 10.8% for deceased donor allografts. The authors concluded that aLDLT increased the capacity for transplantation of stable patients awaiting transplantation without an increased incidence of primary nonfunction and excellent results, but did not significantly impact waitlist mortality (77).

Retrospective data from the A2ALL cohort were presented by Olthoff at the Annual Meeting of the American Surgical Association in 2005: Outcomes of 385 aLDLT performed at nine centers were included. Analysis included 35 donor, recipient, and postoperative variables that were examined by Cox regression modeling to identify risk factors for graft failure. Overall one-year graft survival was 81%, with a 13% incidence of graft failure within the initial 90 days following aLDLT. Complications mirrored existing literature. Older recipient age and length of cold ischemia were the only significant predictors of graft failure by multivariate analysis (86).

The "surgical learning curve" was expressly studied within their analysis. While addressed indirectly by previous authors, Olthoff et al. demonstrated a learning threshold between 10 and 20 procedures with a significantly lower risk of graft failure among centers with a total experience exceeding 20 procedures (86). Later single-center data from Pomfret demonstrated very similar findings (87). While the exact threshold certainly varies among individuals and transplant centers, there is little doubt that repetitive procedures performed by dedicated individuals improve outcomes. This has led to the development of separate standards for UNOS approval of centers wishing to perform LDLT. In its first year of implementation, results of this experience requirement and review and approval process cannot be assessed.

Adult-to-adult living donor liver transplantation was first performed in Europe by Broelsch at Essen in 1998 (88). Broelsch later summarized European aLDLT outcomes by reporting the activity of 11 centers in eight countries performing 105 pediatric and 123 adult living donations. Of the 123 aLDLT, 111 were right lobe allografts (88). The reporting period spanned from 1996 through 2000, during which 2,055 adult transplant procedures were performed; aLDLT represented approximately 6% of the total. Crude recipient and allograft survival were 86% and 83%, respectively, with an observed 14.6% incidence of recipient biliary complications. Other recipient complications were not reported; however, Broelsch did report a European donor death and an overall 30% incidence of donor complications, subclassified as "minor" (14%)

Table 4
Living Donor Liver Transplantation in Europe

Center	Author	Year	N	Recip	Graft	Comp
France(90)	Boillot	2003	88	92%	85%	32%
Essen (89)	Malago	2003	74	79%	75%	30%
Moscow (91)	Gautier	2003	35	100%	97%	37%
Bornova (92)	Tokat	2001	20	75%	75%	75%
Paris (93)	Azoulay	2001	7	100%	85%	42%
Barcelona (94)	Goyet	2001	7	71%	71%	42%
Essen (83)	Malago	2001	43	75%	63%	N/A

Recip = recipient one-year survival; Graft = graft one-year survival; Comp = incidence of complications.

and "major" (17%) (88, 89). These data are in agreement with literature from individual centers (Table 4).

While overall results from Europe and North America are excellent, the recorded incidence of allograft-related complications and utilization among patients with a lower disease severity score at transplantation mirror the practice of extended-donor criteria deceased donor transplantation (EDC).

Inclusion of aLDLT as an EDC allograft is supported through data on allocation, probability of a complication, and risk associated with immediate graft function. EDC and aLDLT allocation occur at the transplant center and are optimal among candidates who do not suffer from acute decompensation of chronic liver disease or fulminant hepatic failure. ALDLT outcomes do not meet expectations of optimal deceased donors (86). Specifically, the incidence of technical complications is higher among aLDLT recipients, and graft survival, when applied to patients in urgent medical need of transplantation, is inferior (95). Poor outcomes in high-urgency recipients has led to recommendations by the New York State Department of Health to restrict aLDLT from patients suffering from fulminant hepatic failure or a Model for End-stage Liver Disease (MELD) score greater than 25.

As aLDLT recipients reflect a highly select group with relatively low MELD scores at transplantation, the most frequent complication leading to aLDLT recipient mortality is allograft dysfunction. Limited application and a higher observed frequency of technical complications create a higher assumed risk for the aLDLT recipient when compared to standard-criteria deceased donor allografts; however, allocation of standard-criteria allografts to potential aLDLT recipients is unlikely.

Adult-to-adult LDLT recipients and donors each assume increased risk to facilitate early transplantation and avoid the morbidity and mortality associated with waiting: a rationale identical to the utilization of EDC. Indeed, pursuing aLDLT may even offer a survival *advantage* when analyzed as an intent-to-treat cohort with candidates who do not have a potential living donor (70).

Living Donor Liver Transplantation in Asia

The evolution of aLDLT has been notably different in Asia, where traditional religious, emotional, and historical ideologies have created significant obstacles to deceased donation (96). The reported annual incidence of brain-death donation remains as low as 0.5 per million population (97) despite legislation for deceased donor-organ retrieval (98, 99). Transplant programs throughout Asia extended living donation to adults as a matter of necessity. To date, successful aLDLT series have been reported in China, Taiwan, Hong Kong, Japan, and Korea. The Shinshu University in Japan initiated the first successful adult LDLT in 1993 using a left lobe allograft (38). Utilization of a right lobe allograft was first described by Habib and Tanaka of Kyoto in 1995; they were attempting to harvest a left lobe for living donor liver transplantation when they discovered anatomical considerations favored a right lobe hepatectomy. Inomata reported a 77% survival rate in the Kyoto initial series of 26 right lobe allografts (84), while Todo of Hokkaido University reported an 80% actual allograft survival in the initial series of 21 right lobe allografts (96). Regional summary data have been published (100–102) that agree with individual center data (Table 5).

Unlike the Western practice of aLDLT, extensive data on left as well as right lobe allografts exist in Asia. These data demonstrate similar

Table 5
Living Donor Liver Transplantation in Asia

Center	Author	Year	N	Recip	Graft	Comp
Hong Kong (82)	Lo	2004	100	92%	90%	38%
New Delhi (103)	Rajasekar	2003	10	100%	60%	30%
Tokyo (104)	Hirata	2002	90	92%	N/A	>20%
Seoul (105)	Lee	2001	157	87%	87%	25%
Matsumoto (106)	Hashikura	2001	38	85%	N/A	16%
Sapporo (107)	Furukawa	2001	14	85%	N/A	14%
Okayama (108)	Inagaki	2001	10	N/A	N/A	40%
Tokyo (109)	Kawasaki	1998	13	84%	84%	8%

outcomes to limited Western data, with a higher incidence of small-for-size syndrome, graft failure, and recipient complications (both biliary and vascular) than right lobe allograft recipients (39, 110–112). The University of Hong Kong Medical Center introduced the utilization of extended right lobe allografts in aLDLT in 1996 in an attempt to overcome inadequate allograft volume and positional problems encountered with the smaller left lobe allografts. Lo reported the first series of seven aLDLT performed with extended right lobe allografts in patients with acute or fulminant hepatic failure (43). This study reported recipient and allograft survival of 86%, which was significantly better than left lobe allograft outcomes; however, the incidence of recipient complications exceeded 30%. Recipient complications included sepsis and hemorrhage from segment IV necrosis, hepatic vein thrombosis, anastomotic biliary leaks, and pancreatitis. After making several technical modifications, a revised series of 22 patients undergoing aLDLT using an extended right lobe allograft demonstrated excellent results with low donor morbidity (44).

Adult-to-Adult Living Donor Liver Transplantation Outcomes When Applied to a Specific Indication

HEPATITIS C

End-stage liver disease secondary to hepatitis C is the leading indication for liver transplantation in the United States, accounting for approximately 40% of the current recipient population. Early concerns with respect to the effect of liver regeneration upon viral replication led to the cautious application of aLDLT within HCV-positive recipients. Gaglio et al. reported an increased incidence of fibrosing cholestatic hepatitis C among aLDLT recipients in a small series with similar data reported by other groups (113). However, well-controlled single-center studies as well as data from the NIH A2ALL study clearly indicate no difference in the incidence and severity of HCV recurrence between aLDLT after the initial 20 cases and deceased whole-organ recipients (114, 114a). In an analysis of aLDLT HCV recipients utilizing protocol biopsies over a four-year follow-up period, Shiffman et al. reported no difference in hepatic inflammation or fibrosis (115). This opens a very important avenue in the treatment of patients with HCV who have well-compensated liver disease and a potential living donor, as it affords the opportunity to maximize viral eradication therapy. If viral eradication is achieved, aLDLT could then proceed with an ~20% chance of HCV recurrence (116).

The Achilles heel of aLDLT application for HCV is the development of a biliary complication. It is likely that early reports of increased viral recurrence among aLDLT recipients were the result of technical complications encountered with the procedure, particularly biliary complications, which created a pro-inflammatory condition within the recipient and stimulated viral replication. It can also hamper early diagnosis of significant recurrent HCV. These reports all reflected data derived during the "surgical learning curve," where the overall incidence of complications was higher and their effective medical management in evolution. However, biliary complications remain a constant threat and can be expected to subvert antiviral therapy and accelerate viral pathology. This is particularly relevant for the potential aLDLT recipient who is unable to tolerate or does not respond to antiviral therapy. When faced with this clinical dilemma, it may be prudent to postpone transplantation to a higher MELD (>15) and consider the application of another EDC allograft with a lower risk profile.

Hepatocellular Carcinoma (HCC)

Living donation has been advocated in the setting of hepatocellular carcinoma. Indeed, typical recipients have little or no signs of end-stage liver failure, with very low physiological MELD scores. Current allocation practice in the United States assigns priority for patients diagnosed with HCC who fulfill the "Milan" criteria reported by Mazzaferro (117). Select regions have extended prioritization to criteria reported by Yao et al. by local arrangement (118). While HCC appears to be the ideal indication for aLDLT, current data are inconclusive with respect to this practice. Multiple single-center reports have demonstrated equivalent outcomes of aLDLT and deceased donor whole-organ transplantation; however, the outcomes reported by Mazzaferro and Yao have not been prospectively validated utilizing aLDLT. Furthermore, recent SRTR and multicenter data from the A2ALL study as well as matched cohort studies by Thuluvath and Lo suggest a higher incidence of HCC recurrence among aLDLT recipients for all stages of disease (95, 119). However, potential increases in posttransplant recurrence must be balanced against decreased waiting-list dropout from tumor progression. Consideration of aLDLT for tumors too large to be accepted as an indication for transplantation (e.g., Stage IV disease with portal vein invasion) should only be performed in the setting of an institutional review board–approved investigational protocol.

Paramount to optimizing aLDLT in the setting of HCC is to capitalize on its advantage as an elective procedure. Gondolesi reported the largest U.S. experience of aLDLT for HCC, including 36 patients transplanted for tumors within and outside the Mazzaferro criteria (120). In this study, mean waiting time for aLDLT recipients was 62 days versus 459 days for deceased donor recipients. ALDLT affords the opportunity for aggressive antitumor therapy to complement traditional loco-regional therapy or investigational neoadjuvant chemotherapy for patients outside recognized criteria for transplantation. Furthermore, in the large subgroup of HCC recipients co-infected with HCV, antiviral therapy can be optimized, yielding the highest chance for viral eradication prior to transplantation. This is a very significant clinical achievement, as SRTR data demonstrate significantly lower HCC recurrence among HCV-positive recipients with a negative viral load at transplantation.

DISCUSSION

The application of aLDLT within North America has remained stable at approximately 4% of annual liver transplants performed since 2001. Factors contributing to the plateau in aLDLT include an improved deceased donor allograft allocation system, increased utilization of expanded-donor criteria deceased donor allografts, improved awareness of surgical risk with respect to physiological MELD, and highly publicized donor deaths. While not increasing in frequency, aLDLT remains an attractive surgical option for highly selected patients and will continue to be performed for the foreseeable future. Indeed, the plateau in performance of aLDLT may be the natural evolution of the procedure until further breakthroughs in the biology of hepatic regeneration or the eradication of hepatitis C provides a stimulus for further expansion.

At present, aLDLT is best applied within the context of an overall EDC program. As with any EDC allograft, there are certain performance strengths and weaknesses. Optimal results are achieved when one plays to the strengths of the procedure; namely, the ability to predict transplantation and premium parenchyma quality. Transplantation as an elective procedure opens new therapeutic avenues that significantly impact a risk–benefit analysis and may justify earlier transplantation with a modestly increased short-term risk. Furthermore, optimal parenchyma quality without an additional theoretical risk of disease transmission is never encountered within EDC except with aLDLT grafts. Therefore, aLDLT becomes the preferred allograft for cholestatic disorders, especially in older children and young adults who are particularly underserved by MELD.

	LDLT	*EDC DDLT*	*Standard DDLT*
Waiting time	Shortest, as needed	Shorter, variable	Longest, variable
Waiting list mortality	Minimal	Intermediate	Highest
Graft quality	Excellent, but reduced size	Variable	Better, but variable
Post-operative morbidity	Increased short-term	Increased short-term and/or long-term	Lowest
Advantages	Shortest waiting time, control of timing of OLT	Shorter waiting time, no donor risk	Improved graft quality and no donor risk
Disadvantages	Donor risk, increase in perioperative complications	Increased risk of immediate graft dysfunction or donor transmitted disease, variable waiting time	Waiting list mortality, increased MELD at transplant, variable waiting time

REFERENCES

1. Renz JF, Busuttil RW. Adult-to-adult living-donor liver transplantation: A critical analysis. *Semin Liver Dis* 2000; 20(4): 411–24.
2. Trotter J, et al. Adult-to-adult transplantation of the right hepatic lobe from a living donor. *N Engl J Med* 2002; 346(14): 1074–82.
3. Russo M, Brown R. Adult living donor liver transplantation. *Am J Transpl* 2004; 4: 458–65.
4. Emond J, Samstein B, Renz J. A critical evaluation of hepatic resection in cirrhosis: Optimizing patient selection and outcomes. *World J Surg* 2005; 29(2): 124–30.
5. Emond JC, Renz JF. Surgical anatomy of the liver and its application to hepatobiliary surgery and transplantation. *Semin Liver Dis* 1994; 14(2): 158–68.
6. Emond JC, et al. Functional analysis of grafts from living donors. Implications for the treatment of older recipients. *Ann Surg* 1996; 224(4): 544–52; disc 552–4.
7. Kiuchi T, et al. Impact of graft size mismatching on graft prognosis in liver transplantation from living donors. *Transplantation* 1999; 67(2): 321–7.

8. Tanaka K, et al. Surgical techniques and innovations in living related liver transplantation. *Ann Surg* 1993; 217(1): 82–91.

9. Ozaki C, et al. Vascular reconstruction in living-related liver transplantation. *Transpl Proc* 1994; 26(1): 167–8.

10. Kuang AA, et al. Decreased mortality from technical failure improves results in pediatric liver transplantation. *Arch Surg* 1996; 131(8): 887–92; disc 892–3.

11. Heffron TG, et al. Biliary complications in pediatric liver transplantation. A comparison of reduced-size and whole grafts. *Transplantation* 1992; 53(2): 391–5.

12. Reichert PR, et al. Biliary complications of reduced-organ liver transplantation. *Liver Transpl Surg* 1998; 4(5): 343–9.

13. Kawasaki S, et al. Liver regeneration in recipients and donors after transplantation. *Lancet* 1992; 339(8793): 580–1.

14. Nakagami M, et al. Patterns of restoration of remnant liver volume after graft harvesting in donors for living related liver transplantation. *Transpl Proc* 1998; 30(1): 195–9.

15. Renz J, et al. Changing faces of liver transplantation: Partial-liver grafts for adults. *J Hepatobil Pancr Surg* 2003; 10(1): 31–44.

16. Renz JF, et al. Donor selection limits use of living-related liver transplantation. *Hepatology* 1995; 22(4 Pt 1): 1122–6.

17. Sterneck M, et al. Evaluation and morbidity of the living liver donor in pediatric liver transplantation. *Transpl Proc* 1995; 27(1): 1164–5.

18. Morimoto T, et al. Donor safety in living related liver transplantation. *Transpl Proc* 1995; 27(1): 1166–9.

19. Ohkohchi N, et al. Complications and treatments of donors and recipients in living-related liver transplantation. *Transpl Proc* 1998; 30(7): 3218–20.

20. Tojimbara T, et al. Analysis of postoperative liver function of donors in living-related liver transplantation: Comparison of the type of donor hepatectomy. *Transplantation* 1998; 66(8): 1035–9.

21. Grewal H, et al. Complications in 100 living-liver donors. *Ann Surg* 1998; 228(2): 214–9.

22. Kadry Z, McCormack L, Clavien P-A. Should living donor liver transplantation be part of every liver transplant program? *J Hepatol* 2005; 43: 32–7.

23. Renz J, Roberts J. Long-term complications of living donor liver transplantation. *Liver Transpl* 2000; 6(6): 73–6.

24. Middleton P, et al. Living donor liver transplantation—Adult donor outcomes: A systematic review. *Liver Transpl* 2006; 12: 24–30.

25. Smith B. Segmental liver transplantation from a living donor. *J Pediatr Surg* 1969; 4: 126–32.

26. Raia S, Nery J, Mies S. Liver transplantation from live donors. *Lancet* 1989; 2: 497.

27. Zitelli BJ, et al. Pediatric liver transplantation: Patient evaluation and selection, infectious complications, and life-style after transplantation. *Transpl Proc* 1987; 19(4): 3309–16.

28. Broelsch CE, et al. Liver transplantation with reduced-size donor organs. *Transplantation* 1988; 45(3): 519–24.

29. Strong RW, et al. Successful liver transplantation from a living donor to her son. *N Engl J Med* 1990; 322(21): 1505–7.

30. Broelsch CE, et al. Liver transplantation in children from living related donors. Surgical techniques and results. *Ann Surg* 1991; 214(4): 428–37; disc 437–9.
31. Renz J, et al. Split-liver transplantation: A review. *Am J Transpl* 2003; 3(11): 1323–35.
32. Roberts J, et al. The influence of graft type on outcomes after pediatric liver transplantation. *Am J Transpl* 2004; 4: 373–7.
33. Abt P, et al. Survival among pediatric liver transplant recipients: Impact of segmental grafts. *Liver Transpl* 2004; 10(10): 1287–93.
34. Harper A, Taranto S, Edwards E. The OPTN waiting list, 1988–2001. *Clin Transpl* 2002; pp. 79–92.
35. Brown R, et al. Liver and intestine transplantation. Am J Transpl 2004; 4(Suppl 9): 81–92.
36. Couinaud C. *Le Foie: Etudes Anatomiques et Chirurgicales.* 1957; Paris: Masson.
37. Bismuth H. Surgical anatomy and anatomical surgery of the liver. *World J Surg* 1982; 6: 3–9.
38. Makuuchi M, et al. Donor hepatectomy for living related partial liver transplantation. *Surgery* 1993; 113(4): 395–402.
39. Miller CM, et al. One hundred nine living donor liver transplants in adults and children: A single-center experience. *Ann Surg* 2001; 234(3): 301–12.
40. Habib N, Tanaka K. Living-related liver transplantation in adult recipients: A hypothesis. *Clin Transpl* 1995; 9(1): 31–4.
41. Wachs ME, et al. Adult living donor liver transplantation using a right hepatic lobe. *Transplantation* 1998; 66(10): 1313–6.
42. Lo C, et al. Extending the limit on the size of adult recipient in living donor liver transplantation using extended right lobe graft. *Transplantation* 1997; 63(10): 1524–8.
43. Lo C, et al. Adult-to-adult living donor liver transplantation using extended right lobe grafts. *Ann Surg* 1997; 226(3): 261–9.
44. Fan S, Lo C, Liu C. Technical refinement in adult-to-adult living donor liver transplantation using right lobe graft. *Ann Surg* 2000; 231(1): 126–31.
45. Pomfret E. Early and late complications in the right-lobe adult living donor. *Liver Transpl* 2003; 9(10 Suppl 2): S45–S49.
46. Pomfret E, et al. Liver regeneration and surgical outcome in donors of right-lobe liver grafts. *Transplantation* 2003; 76(1): 5–10.
47. ASTS. American Society of Transplant Surgeons' position paper on adult-to-adult living donor liver transplantation. *Liver Transpl* 2000; 6(8): 15–7.
48. Shapiro R, Adams M. Ethical issues surrounding adult-to-adult living donor liver transplantation. *Liver Transpl* 2000; 6 (Suppl 2): 77–80.
49. Cronin DN, Millis J, Siegler M. Transplantation of liver grafts from living donors into adults—Too much, too soon. *N Engl J Med* 2001; 344(21): 1633–7.
50. Malago M, et al. Ethical considerations and rationale of adult-to-adult living donor liver transplantation. *Liver Transpl* 2001; 7(10): 921–7.
51. Caplan A. Proceed with caution: Live living donation of lobes of liver for transplantation. *Liver Transpl* 2001; 7(6): 494–5.
52. National Institutes of Health. http://www.nih-a2all.org, 2004.
53. Trotter JF, et al. Right hepatic lobe donation for living donor liver transplantation: Impact on donor quality of life. *Liver Transpl* 2001; 7(6): 485–93.

54. Beavers K, et al. The living donor experience: Donor health assessment and outcomes after living donor liver transplantation. *Liver Transpl* 2001; 7(11): 943–7.
55. Beavers K, Sandler R, Shrestha R. Donor morbidity associated with right lobectomy for living donor liver transplantation to adult recipients: A systematic review. *Liver Transpl* 2002; 8(2): 110–7.
56. Verbesey J, et al. Living donor adult liver transplantation: A longitudinal study of the donor's quality of life. *Am J Transpl* 2005; 5(11): 2770–7.
57. Beavers K, Cassara J, Shrestha R. Practice patterns for long-term follow-up of adult-to-adult right lobectomy donors at U.S. transplantation centers. *Liver Transpl* 2003; 9(6): 645–8.
58. Walter M, et al. Psychosocial stress of living donors after living donor liver transplantation. *Transpl Proc* 2002; 34(8): 3291–2.
59. Marcos A, et al. Single-center analysis of the first 40 adult-to-adult living donor liver transplants using the right lobe. *Liver Transpl* 2000; 6(3): 296–301.
60. Todo S. Adult-to-adult living donor liver transplantation: The Japanese experience. In *Controversies in Transplantation*. 2000; Breckenridge, CO.
61. Testa G, Malago M, Broelsch CE. Living-donor liver transplantation in adults. *Langenbecks Arch Surg* 1999; 384(6): 536–43.
62. Lo C. Complications and long-term outcome of living liver donors: A survey of 1508 cases in five Asian centers. *Transplantation* 2003; 75: S12–S15.
63. Yamaoka Y, et al. Safety of the donor in living-related liver transplantation—An analysis of 100 parental donors. *Transplantation* 1995; 59(2): 224–6.
64. Malago M, et al. Living related liver transplantation: 36 cases at the University of Hamburg. *Transpl Proc* 1994; 26(6): 3620–1.
65. Strong RW. Whither living donor liver transplantation? *Liver Transpl Surg* 1999; 5(6): 536–8.
66. Shaw B. Where monsters hide. *Liver Transpl* 2001; 7: 928–32.
67. Simmons R, Klein S, Simmons R. *Gift of Life: The Social and Psychological Impact of Organ Transplantation*. 1977; New York: Wiley.
68. Diaz G, et al. Donor health assessment after living-donor liver transplantation. *Ann Surg* 2002; 236(1): 120–6.
69. Bay W, Hebert L. The living donor in kidney transplantation. *Ann Intern Med* 1987; 106: 719–27.
70. Russo M, et al. Impact of adult living donor liver transplantation on waiting time survival in candidates listed for liver transplantation. *Am J Transpl* 2004; 4(3): 427–31.
71. United Network for Organ Sharing. http://www.UNOS.org, 2004.
72. Bak T, et al. Adult-to-adult living donor liver transplantation using right-lobe grafts: Results and lessons learned from a single-center experience. *Liver Transpl* 2001; 7(8): 680–6.
73. Humar A. Donor and recipient outcomes after adult living donor liver trasnplantation. *Liver Transpl* 2003; 9: S42–S44.
74. Abt P, et al. Allograft survival following adult-to-adult living donor liver transplantation. *Am J Transpl* 2004; 4: 1302–7.
75. Miller C. Living donor liver transplantation. *Transpl Proc* 2003; 35(3): 964–5.
76. Ghobrial R, et al. Donor and recipient outcomes in right lobe adult living donor liver transplantation. *Liver Transpl* 2002; 8(10): 901–9.

77. Fishbein T, et al. Analysis of 50 consecutive right lobe liver transplants from living donors. In *Proc. Joint Meeting of International Liver Transplantation Society, European Liver Transplantation Association, and Liver Intensive Care Group of Europe*. 2001.

78. Goldstein MJ, et al. Analysis of failure in living donor liver transplantation: Differential outcomes in children and adults. *World J Surg* 2003; 27: 356–64.

79. Fair J, et al. Adult-to-adult living donor liver transplantation using right lobe: Single center experience. In *Proc. the Joint American Transplant Meeting*. 2001; Chicago.

80. Grewal H, et al. Surgical technique for right lobe adult living donor liver transplantation without venovenous bypass or portocaval shunting and with duct-to-duct biliary reconstruction. *Ann Surg* 2001; 233: 502–8.

81. Marcos A, et al. Right lobe living donor liver transplantation. *Transplantation* 1999; 68(6): 798–803.

82. Lo C, et al. Lessons learned from one hundred right lobe living donor liver transplants. *Ann Surg* 2004; 240(1): 151–8.

83. Malago M, et al. Living donor liver transplantation at the University of Essen. In *Proc. Joint Meeting of the International Liver Transplantation Society, European Liver Transplantation Association, and Liver Intensive Care Group of Europe*. 2001.

84. Inomata Y, et al. Right lobe graft in living donor liver transplantation. In *Proc. American Society of Transplant Surgeons*. 1999.

85. Brown R, et al. A survey of liver transplantation from living adult donors in the United States. *N Engl J Med* 2003; 348(9): 818–25.

86. Olthoff K, et al. Outcomes of 385 adult-to-adult living donor liver transplant recipients: A report from the A2ALL consortium. *Ann Surg* 2005; 242(3): 314–25.

87. Pomposelli J, et al. Improved survival after liver donor adult liver transplantation using right lobe grafts: Program experience and lessons learned. *Am J Transpl* 2006; 6(3): 589–98.

88. Broelsch CE, et al. Living donor liver transplantation in adults: Outcome in Europe. *Liver Transpl* 2000; 6(6 Suppl 2): S64–S65.

89. Malago M, et al. Right living donor transplantation: An option for adult patients: Single institution experience with 74 patients. *Ann Surg* 2003; 238(6): 853–62.

90. Boillot O, et al. Initial French experience in adult-to-adult living donor liver transplantation. *Transpl Proc* 2003; 35: 962–3.

91. Gautier S. Living donor liver transplantation in Russia. *Transpl Proc* 2003; 35: 957.

92. Tokat Y, et al. New frontiers: Adult to adult living donor liver transplantation, single center experience from Turkey. *Transpl Proc* 2001; 33(7–8): 3458–60.

93. Azoulay D, et al. Adult to adult living-related liver transplantation. The Paul-Brousse Hospital preliminary experience. *Gastroenterol Clin Biol* 2001; 25(8–9): 773–80.

94. Garcia-Valdecasas J, et al. Adult living donor liver transplantation. In *Proc. Joint Meeting of the International Liver Transplantation Society, European Liver Transplant Association, and the Liver Intensive Care Group of Europe*. 2001.

95. Thuluvath P, Yoo H. Graft and patient survival after adult live donor liver transplantation compared to a matched cohort who received a deceased donor transplantation. *Liver Transpl* 2004; 10(10): 1263–8.

96. Todo S, et al. Living donor liver transplantation in adults: Outcome in Japan. *Liver Transpl* 2000; 6: S66–S72.

97. de Villa VH, et al. Split liver transplantation in Asia. *Transpl Proc* 2001; 33(1–2): 1502–3.

98. Watts J. Concept of brain death to be accepted in South Korea. *Lancet* 1998; 352: 1996.

99. Gutierrez E. Japan's House of Representatives passes brain-death bill. *Lancet* 1997; 349: 1304.

100. Chen C, et al. Living-donor liver transplantation: 12 years of experience in Asia. *Transplantation* 2003; 75: S6–S11.

101. Chen C. Living donor liver transplantation: Experience from Asian countries. In *Proc. International Symposium on Living Donor Organ Transplantation.* 2004.

102. Sugawara Y, Makuuchi M. Advances in adult living donor liver transplantation: A review based on reports from the 10th anniversary of the Adult-to-Adult Living Donor Liver Transplantation Meeting in Tokyo. *Liver Transpl* 2004; 10(6): 715–20.

103. Rajasekar M, et al. Adult-to-adult living donor right lobe liver transplantation: The first series in India. *Transpl Proc* 2003; 35: 70–1.

104. Hirata M, Sugawara Y, Makuuchi M. Living-donor liver transplantation at Tokyo University. *Clin Transpl* 2002; pp. 215–219.

105. Lee S, et al. 157 adult-to-adult living donor liver transplantation. *Transpl Proc* 2001; 33(1–2): 1323–5.

106. Hashikura Y, et al. Long-term results of living-related donor liver graft transplantation: A single-center analysis of 110 transplants. *Transplantation* 2001; 72(1): 95–9.

107. Furukawa H, et al. What is the limit of graft size for successful living donor liver transplantation in adults? *Transpl Proc* 2001; 33(1–2): 1322.

108. Inagaki M, et al. Analysis of donor complications in living donor liver transplantation. *Transpl Proc* 2001; 33(1–2): 1386–7.

109. Kawasaki S, et al. Living related liver transplantation in adults. *Ann Surg* 1998; 227(2): 269–74.

110. Strong R, Fawcett J, Lynch S. Living-donor and split-liver transplantation in adults: Right- versus left-sided grafts. *J Hepatobil Pancr Surg* 2003; 10(1): 5–10.

111. Soejima Y, et al. Outcome analysis in adult-to-adult living donor liver transplantation using the left lobe. *Liver Transpl* 2003; 9(6): 581–6.

112. Sugawara Y, et al. Living-donor liver transplantation in adults: Tokyo University experience. *J Hepatobil Pancr Surg* 2003; 10: 1–4.

113. Gaglio P, et al. Increased risk of cholestatic hepatitis C in recipients of grafts from living versus cadaveric liver donors. *Liver Transpl* 2003; 9(10): 1028–35.

114. Guo L, et al. Living donor liver transplantation for hepatitis C-related cirrhosis: No difference in histological recurrence when compared to deceased donor liver transplantation recipients. *Liver Transpl* 2006; 12: 560–65.

114a. Terrault NA, et al. Outcomes in hepatitis C virus-infected recipients of living donor vs. deceased donor liver transplantation. *Liver Transpl* 2007; 13: 122–9.

115. Shiffman M, et al. Histologic recurrence of chronic hepatits C virus in patients after living donor and deceased donor liver transplantation. *Liver Transpl* 2004; 10(10): 1248.

116. Everson G. Treatment of patients with hepatitis C virus on the waiting list. *Liver Transpl* 2003; 9: S90–S94.

117. Mazzaferro V, et al. Liver transplantation for the treatment of small hepatocellular carcinomas in patients with cirrhosis. *N Engl J Med* 1996; 334: 693–9.

118. Yao F, et al. Liver transplantation for hepatocellular carcinoma: Expansion of the tumor size does not adversely impact survival. *Hepatology* 2001; 33(6): 1394–1403.

119. Lo C, et al. The role and limitation of living donor liver transplantation for hepatocellular carcinoma. *Liver Transpl* 2004; 10(3): 440–7.

120. Gondolesi GE, et al. Adult living donor liver transplantation for patients with hepatocellular carcinoma: Extending UNOS priority criteria. *Ann Surg* 2004; 239: 142–9.

5 The Share 15 Rule

Richard B. Freeman, Jr., MD

CONTENTS

Abstract

The equitable allocation of deceased donor livers for transplantation is an important and contentious issue. The institution of liver allocation based on the Model for End-Stage Liver Disease (MELD) score has allowed prioritization to be based on an objective measure of illness. In addition, after institution of the MELD system, policy makers were now able to measure differences among patients, institutions, and geographical areas that are much less influenced by the artificial biases that waiting time introduced. A careful analysis of MELD scores <15 showed that patients face a greater mortality risk from the transplant procedure than from their liver disease without surgery. As a result, the organ allocation policy was changed such that regional sharing is now based on offering organs to candidates with MELD score ≥ 15 before local allocation to patients with MELD scores <15. Since the institution of the "Share 15" policy, the number of transplants performed in patients with high MELD score has increased, while the number of deaths on the transplant list has decreased.

Key Words: Liver transplantation; Organ allocation; Liver allocation; Model for End-Stage Liver Disease

From: *Clinical Gastroenterology: Liver Transplantation: Challenging Controversies and Topics*
Edited by: G. T. Everson and J. F. Trotter, DOI: 10.1007/978-1-60327-028-1_5,
© Humana Press, Totowa, NJ

INTRODUCTION

The national policy in the United States for assigning deceased donor livers to waiting liver transplant candidates depends on two factors: allocation and distribution. Allocation is the method by which a group of waiting candidates is ordered in priority. Distribution defines pools of candidates in increasingly larger geographic areas who are subjected to the allocation rules. Under U.S. policy, when a deceased donor is identified in a given donor service area (DSA), non-emergent candidates waiting at transplant centers served by the Organ Procurement Organization (OPO) covering that DSA (Fig. 1) are ranked first in priority, followed by candidates waiting at centers in the larger geographic Organ Procurement and Transplantation Network (OPTN) Region (Fig. 2), followed by remaining candidates in the rest of the nation (Table1). Within each geographic distribution unit, candidates are ordered by allocation rules. Thus, both allocation rules and geographic sequence play a role in determining which candidate will receive a given deceased donor liver.

Because of the extremely constrained donor resource and the need to strive for equitable allocation, much attention and controversy have been directed toward the geographic variations in the United States (1–3). There is considerable variation in transplantation rates (4), severity of illness at the time of transplant (5), and death rates on the waiting list

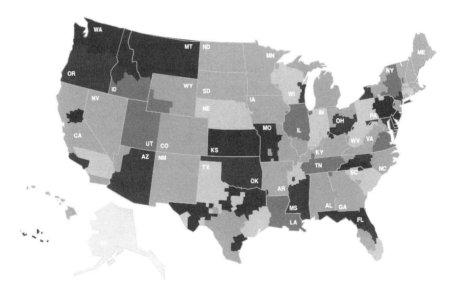

Fig. 1. Donor Service Areas for the 63 Organ Procurement Organizations as of 2003.

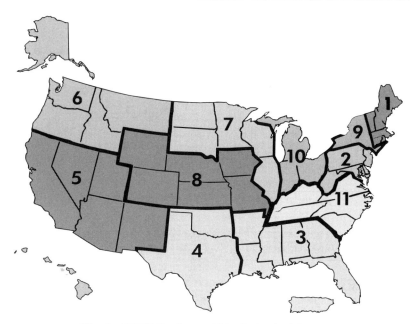

Fig. 2. OPTN Regions within the United States.

(6) among the DSAs and regions. In previous liver allocation policy iterations—when time waiting on the list carried significant weight in determining priority within a DSA—considerable differences in waiting time among the DSAs and Regions fueled the debate regarding the fairness of the system. Many political, institutional, and social forces came to bear on this problem; legislators in Wisconsin, Louisiana, Arizona, and Florida passed laws to preclude the distribution of transplanted organs to residents outside their state (7). In 1997, in response to these controversies, the Department of Health and Human Services issued a draft "Final Rule" regarding organ allocation and distribution, which served to engender even more controversy. In October 1998, Congress delayed implementation of this rule and commissioned the Institute of Medicine (IOM) to study these issues. The IOM report published in 1999 concluded, among other things, that "Creation of organ allocation areas [distribution areas] based on a minimum population of approximately 9 million persons would substantially increase the allocation of organs to patients with more urgent need of transplantation" and that combining geographically contingent DSAs would be the least disruptive method for constructing these new sharing areas (8).

Combining adjacent DSAs, however, proved to be a difficult proposition. In one study where mathematical models were used to examine

Table 1
General Liver Distribution Sequence in the United States

1. Longest-waiting blood type–compatible emergent[1]
    (Status 1) candidate within the local (DSA) area in which
    the donor hospital is located.
2. Longest-waiting blood type–compatible emergent[1]
    (Status 1) candidate within the OPTN Region in which
    the donor hospital is located.
3. Highest-ranking (by prevailing allocation policy[2]),
    non-emergent blood type–compatible candidate within
    the local (DSA) area in which the donor hospital is
    located.
4. Highest-ranking (by prevailing allocation policy[2]),
    non-emergent blood type–compatible candidates within
    the OPTN Region in which the donor hospital is located.
5. Highest-ranking (by prevailing allocation policy[2]),
    non-emergent blood type–compatible candidate within
    the nation.

[1] Emergent: Status 1: Fulminant hepatic failure, primary graft failure,
hepatic artery thrombosis.
[2] Prior to February 2002, this allocation policy was defined as
Status 2A: ICU bound, CTP score $\geq$ 10.
Status 2B: CTP $\geq$ 10 with decompensation, not in ICU.
Status 3: CTP $\geq$ 7.
After February 2002, allocation policy was redefined using
MELD/PELD score.

the effects of combining distribution units, seven different geographical
distribution area configurations were drawn and 17 different allocation
sequences were examined. These models did not reveal any overall improvement in waiting list or transplant outcomes (9). The authors of this
study attributed these results to the fact that many contiguous DSAs
have similar underlying donor and waiting list dynamics. For example,
DSAs in New York and New England each already cover more than 9
million residents, but they have some of the lowest transplantation rates
and highest death rates of all regions in the country (6). Moreover, combining DSAs in the Southeast, where donation rates are relatively high
compared with the number of waiting patients and where waiting times
are already relatively short, would only exacerbate differences. Furthermore, waiting time on the list was determined much more by physician
listing practice behavior than actual intrinsic patient condition, it was
clear that a ranking system based on individual patient characteristics,

not the doctors' behavior, was needed before organs could be directed more precisely to those most in need and not just to those who could wait the longest.

At the time, observers began to appreciate that redrawing organ distribution boundaries was an indirect and imprecise method for directing organs to the candidates with the highest urgency. In order to more directly offer organs to the most appropriate candidates, the definition of need for transplant had to be more patient-centered, explicitly defined, and less subject to observer bias. These realizations provided the impetus to change the system to significantly reduce the influence of waiting time and apply more objective measures of patient disease severity. This was the genesis for implementation of the MELD/PELD system (10), where waiting time was essentially eliminated and a much more objective assessment of patient need as defined by mortality risk was introduced. The MELD/PELD system of allocation more accurately prioritizes patients with higher risks of dying from their liver diseases than the former, more subjective system, that was driven by waiting time/CTP categories. Moreover, after institution of the MELD/PELD algorithm, policy makers were able to measure differences among patients, institutions, and geographical areas with much more objective, patient-based metrics that are much less influenced by the artificial biases that waiting time introduced. After 18 months of experience with the MELD/PELD system, the liver transplant community was able to assess the geographic disparities in liver allocation with more impartiality and was able to provide much more valid estimations of the waiting list and transplantation dynamics.

In December 2003, a wide array of liver transplant community members attended a conference to discuss the early results of the new MELD/PELD system and to address future directions (11). This was a unique event because of the wide participation and, importantly, the amount of objective data available for critical review. Dr. Robert Wolfe from the Scientific Registry for Transplant Recipients (SRTR) described results indicating that, since the initiation of MELD/PELD, most first donor liver offers were occurring for candidates with MELD score <10 (Fig. 3). In addition, he showed that almost half (46%) of the transplants were being performed for candidates with MELD scores <20 at the time of transplantation (Fig. 4) and that, in some DSAs, a significant proportion of transplants were being performed for candidates with MELD score <10 (Fig. 5). From these results, the participants concluded that, under the system prevailing at the time, a significant number of liver grafts were being directed to candidates with low MELD scores, possibly because organ distribution boundaries were preventing the sharing

Offers

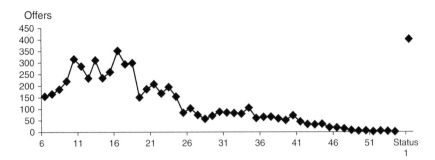

Fig. 3. MELD score at first offer for donors during the period from April 1, 2002 through July 31, 2003. Offers to exceptional candidates excluded. [Adapted from Wolfe, *Liver Transpl* 2004; 10(Suppl 2):A6–A22].

of organs with centers in adjacent DSAs having higher MELD score candidates.

One suggestion put forth at the meeting was to limit entry on the liver waiting list to those candidates with MELD scores of at least 10 or possibly even of 15 or higher. Modeling done with the SRTR Liver Simulated Allocation Model (LSAM) indicated that the number of transplants for higher MELD patients would increase while the number of patients removed for death on the waiting list would decrease (Table 2). Several participants pointed out that the MELD score is an estimate, with confidence intervals such that there is some overlapping of mortality risk estimates (12) and there are some candidates with low MELD scores who can benefit from liver transplantation. Nonetheless, data

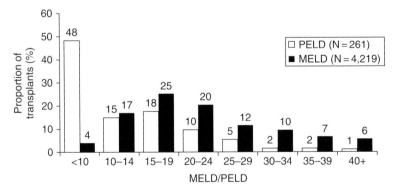

Fig. 4. MELD/PELD score at transplant for deceased donor liver transplants performed during the period from April 1, 2002 through July 31, 2003. [Adapted from Wolfe, *Liver Transpl* 2004; 10(Suppl 2):A6–A22].

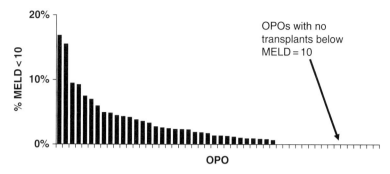

Fig. 5. Proportion of transplants in patients with MELD score < 10 at transplant by OPO. [Adapted from Wolfe, *Liver Transpl* 2004; 10(Suppl 2): A6–A22].

presented at this conference and subsequently published (13) indicated that the vast majority of candidates with MELD scores of 15 or lower face a greater mortality risk from the transplant procedure than from their liver disease without surgery. This combination of pretransplant mortality risk with posttransplant mortality risk into a single calculation has been termed *transplant benefit*. As a result of these deliberations, conferees recommended that the OPTN develop a policy of "regional

Table 2

LSAM Predicted Changes in Number of Transplants and Removals for Death on the Waiting List if Waiting List Entry Was Limited to Patients with MELD Scores ≥ 10 or Limited to Patients with MELD ≥ 15 Compared with the Policy Prevailing at That Time

	Prevailing	*MELD ≥ 10*	*MELD ≥ 15*
Deaths			
Waitlist	860	840	781
Posttransplant	164	165	178
Total	1,024	1,005	959
Transplants			
MELD 0–9	131	0	0
MELD 10–18	759	805	553
MELD 19–24	789	855	994
MELD 25–40	630	659	784
Status 1	251	262	290
Total	2,560	2,581	2,621

Source: Adapted from Wolfe, *Liver Transpl* 2004; 10(Suppl 2):A6–A22.

1. Local Status 1
2. OPTN Region Status 1
3. Local (DSA)   MELD ≥ 15
4. OPTN Region MELD ≥ 15
5. Local (DSA)   MELD < 15
6. OPTN Region   MELD < 15
7. National   All MELD

Fig. 6. Share 15 liver distribution sequence for adult donor liver.

sharing to MELD score greater than or equal to 15 before local allocation to patients with MELD scores less than 15" (11).

The OPTN programmed and initiated this new, so-called Share-15, policy in January 2005 (Fig. 6). The intent of this policy is to limit the transplantation of patients with the lower MELD scores that are indicative of better survival without a transplant by requiring that organs can be used for these less ill patients only after all other patients in the OPTN Region with MELD score of at least 15 have had the opportunity to accept such an offer. Thus, this policy does not completely preclude transplantation of these patients, but it requires that all other candidates more likely to benefit from transplant have had their opportunity first. Although this new policy does not redraw any distribution unit boundaries, it effectively broadens them by requiring organs to be shared among DSAs when there are no candidates possessing MELD scores indicating a benefit for transplantation listed at a center in the DSA in which the organ was procured.

One of the important aspects of this policy, a quality that would not be possible where transplant priority is defined by more subjective and potentially malleable variables, is that it is patient-based and not driven by center, political, socioeconomic, or other less desirable forces. In addition, those who argue to keep organs within a DSA (or State or Region) to serve their own patients first even if they do not have a demonstrable benefit as measured by a MELD score less than 15 are not acting in the best interest of their patients. Such a patient-based approach also makes it difficult to justify obligatory state laws, since retaining organs within a state for the purpose of providing transplants to state residents with low MELD scores first, actually imposes a higher mortality risk with a transplant than they would face without one.

Comparing liver transplantation dynamics from January 2004 through August 2004 (the year prior to implementation of the Share 15 rule) with the corresponding time period under Share 15 (January 2005–August 2005), we see an increase in the number of transplants

Table 3
Number of Deceased Donor Liver Transplants Before and After Share 15 Rule,
by Type of Share

	Before Share 15 (%)	After Share 15 (%)	Total (%)
Local	2,416 (71.4)	2,565 (69.7)	4,981 (70.5)
Regional	779 (23.0)	833 (22.6)	1,612 (22.8)
National	187 (5.5)	284 (7.7)	471 (6.7)

performed at every distribution unit designation and no change in the proportion of transplants performed at the local, regional, and national levels (Table 3). The removal rate for death or too sick (Fig. 7) has decreased for the lower MELD patients and has remained essentially unchanged for the MELD $\geq$ 15 candidates. When we stratify by MELD score at removal, we see an increase in the number of transplants performed in the upper two MELD score deciles and a decrease in the lower MELD score categories, with slight decreases in the removals for death or too sick in the higher MELD score strata (Fig. 8). In addition, the MELD score at transplant has increased within the DSAs, but there does not appear to be a net shift in organs across DSAs as a result of the Share 15 policy. These results indicate that there has not been a

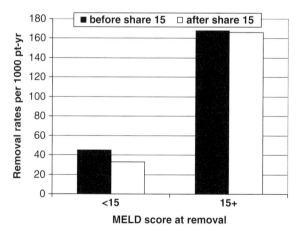

Fig. 7. Removal rates for death on the waiting list comparing the period from January 12, 2004, through August 31, 2004 (before Share 15), with same period during 2005 (after Share 15). Adults only, with match MELD score used for MELD at removal calculations. Based on OPTN data as of December 2, 2005.

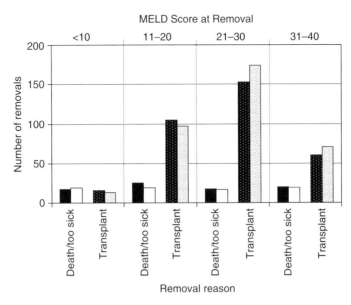

Fig. 8. Reason for removal before and after Share 15 rule stratified by match MELD score at removal, before (■) and after (□) Share-15 rule. Based on OPTN data as of December 2, 2005.

significant redistribution of organs outside the DSA. However, transplant centers appear to be identifying candidates with higher MELD scores for transplant, more transplants are being performed for candidates with higher MELD scores, fewer of these patients are dying on the list, and fewer transplants are being performed for the patients least likely to benefit from transplantation. These very preliminary results suggest that this Share 15 policy has slightly increased the direction of organs to candidates with a higher mortality risk. However, these changes are slight at best, there does not appear to be a significant redistribution of organs, and more results will need to be evaluated to determine if probabilities of transplant have changed for candidates who are sicker.

Future policy developments will further refine criteria for defining need. One can envision possible new policies requiring sharing for additional patient-defined conditions. In fact, data suggesting that the smallest children waiting for livers have the highest mortality risk while waiting (10) have resulted in the adoption of regional sharing for pediatric donors (14). Again, the goal of this policy is to better direct donor organs to those most in need—in this case children with the highest mortality risk. Most importantly, policy must continue to focus on objective patient characteristics for organ allocation and distribution. Redistributing organs because artificial boundaries have highlighted discrepancies can be misguided, because such shifting of organs does not necessarily directly affect the waiting patients. However, patient-based allocation and distribution requires that a transparent system, employing the most objective patient-specific variables, is in place. This is necessary so that policy makers and the public can have a clearer understanding of the dynamics of the organ allocation system, the practice behaviors, and other geopolitical and socioeconomic forces that all affect the outcome of the deceased donor allocation and distribution system.

ACKNOWLEDGMENT

The data analyses presented here were supported in part by Health Resources and Services Administration contract 231-00-0115. The content of this chapter is the responsibility of the authors alone and does not necessarily reflect the views or policies of the U.S. Department of Health and Human Services, nor does mention of trade names, commercial products, or organizations imply endorsement by the U.S. Government.

REFERENCES

1. Norman DJ. Allocation of livers for liver transplantation: Ethics and politics. *Clin Liver Dis* 1997; 1: 281–6.
2. Ellison MD, Edwards LB, Edwards EB, Barker CF. Geographic differences in access to transplantation in the United States. *Transplantation* 2003; 76:1389–94.
3. Schaffer RL 3rd, Kulkami S, Harper A, Millis JM, Cronin DC 2nd. The sickest first? Disparities with model for end-stage liver disease-based organ allocation: One region's experience. *Liver Transpl* 2003; 9:1211–5.
4. Freeman RB, Wiesner RH, Roberts JP, McDiarmid SV, Dykstra D, Merion RM. SRTR report on the state of liver transplantation. Improving liver allocation: MELD and PELD. *Am J Transpl* 2004; 4(Suppl 9):114–31.
5. Trotter JF, Osgood MJ. MELD scores of liver transplant recipients according to size of waiting list. *JAMA* 2004; 291:1871–4.
6. Freeman RB, Edwards EB, Harper AM. Trends in MELD score and transplantation rates under the MELD system. *Hepatology* 2005; 42(Suppl 1):203A.
7. Meckler LA. States fight organ donation policy. AP wire service, July 14, 1998.
8. *Organ Procurement and Transplantation: Assessing Current Policies and the Potential Impact of the DHHS Final Rule.* 1999; Washington, DC: National Academy Press, p. 7.
9. Freeman RB, Harper AM, Edwards EB. Redrawing organ distribution boundaries: Results of a computer-simulated analysis for liver transplantation. *Liver Transpl* 2002; 8:659–66.

10. Freeman RB, Wiesner RH, Harper A, McDiarmid SV, Lake J, Edwards EB, Merion R, Wolfe R, Turcotte J, Teperman L. The new liver allocation system: Moving toward evidence-based transplantation policy. *Liver Transpl* 2002; 8: 851–8.
11. Olthoff KM, Brown RS, DelMonico FL, Freeman RB, McDiarmid SV, Merion RM, Millis JM, Roberts JP, Shaked A, Wiesner RH, Lucey MR. Summary report of a national conference: Evolving concepts in liver allocation in the MELD/PELD era. *Liver Transpl* 2004; 10(Suppl 2):A6–A22.
12. Merion RM. When is a patient too well and when is a patient too sick for a liver transplant? *Liver Transpl* 2004; 10(Suppl 2):S69–S73.
13. Merion RM, Schaubel DE, Dykstra DM, Freeman RB, Port FK, Wolfe RA. The survival benefit of liver transplantation. *Am J Transpl* 2005; 2:307–13.
14. See www.optn.org, policy 3.6.

6 Hepatocellular Carcinoma

Michael A. Zimmerman, MD,
Andrew M. Cameron, MD, PhD,
and R. Mark Ghobrial, MD, PhD

CONTENTS

Abstract

The preferred therapy for patients with end-stage liver disease and hepatocellular carcinoma (HCC) is orthotopic liver transplantation (OLT). The increase in viral hepatitis over the last two decades has led a dramatic increase in the incidence of HCC in the United States and other Western countries. In fact, the number of patients with HCC listed for transplantation will exceed the total number of available donors in the future. Preoperative staging of HCC is

From: *Clinical Gastroenterology: Liver Transplantation: Challenging Controversies and Topics*
Edited by: G. T. Everson and J. F. Trotter, DOI: 10.1007/978-1-60327-028-1_6,
© Humana Press, Totowa, NJ

difficult and frequently understages the extent of disease. There is controversy in the selection of patients with extensive-stage HCC for liver transplantation. In addition, living donor liver transplantation offers expedited transplantation, but ethical issues over the application of this procedure in HCC patients have raised concerns. Prior to transplantation, the two most commonly applied therapies are transarterial chemoembolization (TACE) and radiofrequency ablation (RFA). In properly selected patients, the posttransplantation outcomes are favorable. Finally, the selection of the posttransplantation immunosuppressive protocol may help to reduce HCC recurrence.

Key Words: Hepatocellular carcinoma; Living donor liver transplantation; Transarterial chemoembolization; Radiofrequency ablation; Immunosuppression

INTRODUCTION

Orthotopic liver transplantation (OLT) is the preferred treatment option for patients with end-stage liver disease and hepatocellular carcinoma (HCC). With the global increase in viral hepatitis over the last two decades, the incidence of HCC in the United States and other Western countries is rising dramatically (1). Cirrhosis with concomitant HCC will prove much more common in the next 25 years (2). As such, the number of patients with HCC listed for transplantation will exceed the total number of available donors in the future (3).

Mechanistically, chronic inflammation in the cirrhotic liver promotes a dysplastic field. While hepatocellular cancers tend to be multifocal, involving more than one segment of the liver, many lesions are not anatomically amenable to surgical resection. This is further complicated by underlying liver dysfunction (4). Thus, tumor excision via total hepatectomy at the time of OLT offers the best oncological solution. However, for approximately 15–20% of patients transplanted with HCC, recurrent tumor remains a formidable problem (5–7).

With universal application of the Model for End-Stage Liver Disease (MELD) in 2002 in the United States, patients with HCC are given increased priority on the waiting list. As a result, the number of patients with cancer transplanted in the MELD era has increased threefold (8, 9). The initial experience with OLT for patients with HCC was dismal (10). However, an important experience reported by Mazzaferro and colleagues from Milan chronicled the outcome in a small cohort of patients transplanted for HCC (11). With the introduction of strict selection criteria, an 85% four-year survival was achieved. Conversely, those exceeding these "Milan criteria" had a four-year survival of 50%. These parameters have been adopted by the United Network of Organ Sharing (UNOS) for patients with HCC and are the basis for organ allocation in the United States (12).

As our experience with transplantation for cancer evolves, several controversial areas of clinical management have emerged. While we have seen a significant improvement in long-term outcomes in the last two decades (13), some have advocated expanding the selection criteria in this patient population. Further, as chemotherapy for HCC has no proven benefit (14), loco-regional ablative therapies are increasingly being employed in an attempt to provide a "bridge" to OLT. Similarly, some have advocated hepatic resection in patients with preserved liver function followed by "salvage" OLT in the event of cancer recurrence or liver failure. However, the impact of these strategies on survival after OLT remains unclear. Finally, the true impact of immunosuppression and the optimal treatment of recurrent HCC are controversial.

EXPANDING THE SELECTION CRITERIA FOR TRANSPLANTATION AND HCC

Liver transplantation offers the best chance at long-term survival for patients with HCC and cirrhosis. However, with a severe shortage of cadaveric donors, organ allocation is based on predicted outcomes (15). With the evolution of the surgical approach to HCC, patients can be stratified into three distinct groups. Those with preserved liver function and a resectable tumor should be offered surgical resection. Patients with unresectable lesions and/or severe dysfunction should be considered for transplantation. Currently, no uniform selection criteria are applied internationally. As a result, exactly which patients are listed for transplantation is not firmly established.

OLT and Cadaveric Donation

An early series from the University of Pittsburgh included over 100 patients who underwent OLT for HCC (10). Five-year survival in this cohort was approximately 36%, with tumor recurrence over 40%. Our experience at the University of California, Los Angeles (UCLA) during this time period included 28 patients, with only three living longer than five years (16). Tumor recurrence was nearly 50% in patients living longer than three months. The strict selection criteria introduced by Mazzaferro in 1996 (solitary lesions less than 5 cm, or multiple lesions, not more than three, none exceeding 3 cm) changed the approach to transplantation for HCC. Limiting OLT to patients with small, contained lesions had a dramatic effect on survival and promoted global change in patient selection.

Several studies have since confirmed the positive effect of the "Milan criteria" in different patient populations. Figueras and colleagues from Barcelona reported their experience shortly after the introduction of these parameters (17). Excluding patients without cirrhosis, as well as those with incidental lesions, five-year survival between patients with HCC and those without was no different (68% vs. 71%). Overall tumor recurrence was observed in only 8%. Similar observations were made by other groups (18, 19). The success of this conservative approach has led a number of centers to identify their own criteria for OLT in HCC patients. Iwatsuki and colleagues at the University of Pittsburgh initially defined three factors associated with significantly poor outcome (20). Using tumor size larger than 5 cm, bilobar tumors, and presence of vascular invasion, they calculated a prognostic risk score grading the probability to tumor recurrence. Five-year survival was 100% in patients with a grade 1 and 0% in those with a grade 5.

In 2001, Yao and colleagues from the University of California, San Francisco (UCSF) introduced an expanded criteria: single tumor ≤ 6.5 cm or no more than three tumors, the largest of which ≤ 4.5 cm, and total tumor diameter of ≤ 8 cm (21). Survival at five years was over 70%, with an 11.4% recurrence rate. When applied to patients at a separate center, these criteria revealed similar results. Nearly 400 patients transplanted at the University of Pittsburgh were stratified by pathologic data to within or exceeding the UCSF criteria (15). Five-year survival among the patients meeting these parameters was 67%, with only a 4.5% recurrence rate. A follow-up study by the UCSF group suggests that the San Francisco criteria may serve as a better predictor of acceptable outcome than Milan (22). The authors emphasize that the UCSF parameters do not require the pathologic confirmation of vascular invasion such as the Pittsburgh scoring system.

Based on these observations, proponents of expanding the existing criteria in the United States argue that comparable survival can be achieved with more liberal patient selection (12). Ironically, survival within the "Milan" era may be too good. As OLT offers the only real chance of cure for patients with unresectable lesions, some suggest that the current parameters for patient selection are too restrictive. While there is no unified approach to OLT for HCC internationally, many patients excluded from the cadaveric donor pool may seek viable alternatives including living donor liver transplant (LDLT). Those opposed to expanding the selection criteria argue that tumor characteristics employed to predict outcome (i.e., tumor size, vascular invasion, grade, etc.) can only truly be evaluated pathologically. This information is not completely available preoperatively, making a liberalization of the selection criteria much too risky a proposition (23). With disparities in abdominal imaging, and the lack of reliable tumor markers, expanding the definition of appropriate candidates for OLT may lead to an increase in tumor recurrence and a dramatic reduction in survival.

Living Donor Liver Transplant

Prolonged waiting times and an increasing dropout rate are the major problems with transplantation via cadaveric donation (24). As such, more centers are beginning to offer LDLT to patients with HCC. First performed in the United States in the late 1990s (25), LDLT has rapidly become a viable treatment option for patients with end-stage liver disease (26). The cumulative experience in the United States of 385 adult LDLT recipients includes 60 patients (16%) with HCC (27). Overall, one-year graft survival was 81%, with a 30% incidence of biliary complications and 13% early graft failure. Despite technical issues, the obvious advantage to living donation is the shortened waiting time. Additionally, recipients transplanted electively are generally healthier at the time of surgery. Several reports suggest that survival rates are comparable to cadaveric OLT (28, 29).

The bulk of experience with LDLT for malignancy comes from Asia, where cadaveric donors are rare. A large series from Japan documents 316 LDLT recipients with HCC (29). One- and three-year patient survival are 78% and 69%, respectively. The overall recurrence rate is 12.7%. Interestingly, when the Milan criteria were applied, the three-year recurrence-free survival was 79%. This fell to 52.6% in those exceeding the criteria. Importantly, the three-year recurrence rate for patients outside the Milan criteria was 32.2%, compared to 1.6% in those meeting the criteria. Macrovascular invasion was the most prominent risk factor for recurrence. A recent series from Korea provides a direct comparison of LDLT to cadaveric donor OLT (30). No significant difference was noted in one- or two-year recurrence-free survival between the groups. Not surprisingly, gross vascular invasion, histological differentiation, and tumor size were independent risk factors for recurrence. Overall, the Milan and UCSF inclusion criteria were met by 70% and 77.7% of patients, respectively. When Milan or USCF parameters were met, three-year survival was markedly better, at approximately 90%. These data confirm that the tumor size restrictions imposed by the current selection criteria have a positive impact on the incidence of HCC recurrence. Additionally, these indices are applicable to either cadaveric or living donation. Furthermore, the theoretic concern that tumor recurrence would be accelerated in the context of vigorous liver regeneration after LDLT has not been realized.

Several concerns specific to LDLT and criteria expansion have been raised (23). Primarily, the potential harm to a healthy donor continues to be central to the general argument against living donation. With a general recurrence rate of 10–20%, some question subjecting a healthy individual to such an extensive and invasive procedure that may not provide a reasonable chance at long-term survival for the recipient. Additionally, opponents argue that cancer has a specific psychological burden that may lead to coercion. This may be intensified for recipients with large tumors beyond UNOS criteria. Finally, one has the ethical dilemma of how to proceed if the LDLT graft fails. Should these patients be given consideration for cadaveric OLT?

MARGINAL CADAVERIC DONORS AND HCC

In an effort to expand the existing donor pool, criteria defining an acceptable cadaveric donor are continually being refined. As such, a strict definition of a "marginal donor" has not been established. However, donors at increased risk of primary non-function (PNF), or initial poor function (IPF), are generally considered marginal. Experts in the field agree that while these organs are not optimal, they are a viable alternative to dying on the waiting list for transplantation and should be used where deemed appropriate (31). Factors associated with PNF or IPF include advance donor age, prolonged ischemia time, hypotension, gender mismatch, non-heart-beating donors, and steatosis (32–35). Busuttil and Tanaka commented that ischemia-reperfusion (IR) injury is the root cause of graft dysfunction in marginal organs (31).

Several precautionary measures can be employed that may improve hepatic tolerance to IR, including choosing a healthy recipient and lowering cold ischemic time (CIT). Busuttil and Tanaka recommended that marginal grafts from donors that are over 60 years old, have >30% or <60% steatosis, ICU stay >5 days, or require more than one vasopressor should be maximized by keeping the CIT <8 hours and selecting a good-risk recipient (31). Several centers have reported their experience with marginal grafts. Rocha and colleagues from Brazil documented 148 patients undergoing OLT (36). The rate of marginal donors in this cohort was 61.5% defined by age >55, AST >150 UI/L, bilirubin >2 mg/dL, serum sodium = 150 mEq/L, cardiac arrest, ICU stay >5 days, and moderate to severe macrosteatosis. Survival at six months was 81% for those receiving marginal grafts and 70.7% from ideal donors. These differences were not significant. These findings have been corroborated by other groups (37–39), suggesting that organs from moderately ill donors can safely be used in the face of suboptimal conditions.

Few studies exist that apply the concept of extended criteria donation to patients with HCC. A European series from Sotiropoulos and colleagues documented the success rate of transplantation for recipients with HCC using "livers that nobody wants" (40). Over a three-year period, they accepted and transplanted 10 deceased donor allografts that had been officially rejected on 40 separate occasions by other transplant centers. With a median follow-up of 12 months (range: 5 to 36 months), all patients were alive at the time of publication. While nine of the 10 recipients had a T3 or greater tumor, 50% were beyond Milan criteria. The authors specifically sought to challenge the notion of extending the recipient criteria, as well as using marginal cadaveric donation, in patients with HCC. They argue that the risk–benefit ratio is positive in their experience, as illustrated by a short waiting time (median of 63 days), an acceptable rate of IPF (20%), and 100% patient and graft survival in the short term.

ACCURACY OF PREOPERATIVE STAGING

Within the chronic inflammatory environment of the cirrhotic liver, severe fibrosis, nodular dysplasia, and ultimately invasive cancer represent a pathologic continuum. At present, determining the difference between dysplasia and invasive carcinoma is problematic. Tumor characteristics including size, number of lesions, and anatomical location are the cornerstone to preoperative staging and strongly influence patient management. As such, radiological imaging is routinely employed to make the diagnosis of HCC, as well as quantifying tumor burden and subsequent suitability for transplantation. Unfortunately, the accuracy of preoperative imaging has been called into question.

Most centers employ computed tomography (CT) or magnetic resonance imaging (MRI) to evaluate patients prior to transplant. However, the accuracy of each method in the setting of both cancer and cirrhosis is unclear. An early study by Vogl and colleagues retrospectively reviewed 33 consecutive biphasic CT scans in patients with cirrhosis and HCC prior to either liver resection or OLT (41). Findings on imaging were compared to pathologic specimens. The sensitivity of CT for lesions less than 1 cm was 20%. However, this increased to 100% for lesions greater than 3 cm. Libbrecht et al. compared ultrasound, CT, and MRI in cirrhotic patients with HCC within six months of OLT (42). Interestingly, ultrasound proved to be a crude modality (sensitivity of 40%), as it detected only the largest cancers and was unable to detect dysplastic nodules. The sensitivity of CT and MRI was also poor in detecting dysplastic lesions, at 20% and 27%, respectively. Conversely, the sensitivity of CT and MRI for detecting HCC was 50% and 70%, respectively. The authors concluded that MRI, while far from perfect, is the best tool available for evaluating patients with cirrhosis to identify and/or follow the progression of HCC. Similar findings have been reported by other groups (43).

The inability to accurately assess tumor burden preoperatively results in transplanting an unknown percentage of patients who do not meet the currently accepted selection criteria. In the series by Mazzaferro et al., 13 patients who underwent OLT (27%) were understaged prior to transplant (11). In a report from Japan including 56 patients transplanted for HCC by LDLT, only 21 patients (37.5%) were correctly evaluated for tumor number prior to transplant (44). The remaining 35 patients were incorrectly assessed, with 26 patients understaged. A larger series from Germany made similar observations (40). Over 70% of patients who underwent OLT for cirrhosis and HCC had incorrect measurements of tumor diameter greater than 1 cm. Using either CT or MRI, the sensitivity for lesions between 1 and 2 cm was only 21%. Based on preoperative imaging alone, 14 of 70 patients exceeded the Milan criteria. However, comparing these findings to post-OLT explants, the number of patients outside the criteria increased to 21. Overall, 40% of patients were incorrectly staged. Cumulatively, these data confirm that current imaging techniques are suboptimal in estimating preoperative tumor burden. As a result, some patients will be transplanted who exceed the accepted selection criteria. More importantly, an unknown percentage of patients will be denied OLT based on inaccurate staging.

LOCO-REGIONAL ABLATIVE THERAPY

Transplantation as a therapeutic option in patients with HCC and cirrhosis presents a unique clinical dilemma. As the number of cadaveric donors falls well short of the number of patients on the waiting list, an unknown period of time will pass between listing and OLT. Thus, tumor progression past the accepted criteria may lead to "dropout" from the list for a subset of patients. To date, chemotherapy pre- and postoperatively has not proven effective in patients with HCC (14). As a result, local ablative techniques, including transarterial (TACE) and radiofrequency ablation (RFA), are increasingly being utilized prior to transplant. Theoretically, the induction of tumor necrosis may attenuate progression over time and reduce the rate of patient loss from the waiting list.

A study from UCSF chronicled the dropout rate while on the waiting list in a cohort of 70 patients (45). Overall, 18 patients (22.6%) dropped off the list over approximately 24 months. The cumulative rate of dropout was 7.2% between 0 and 6 months on the list. However, beyond six months, the probability of dropout increased dramatically. At 12, 18, and 24 months, the cumulative probability of dropout was 37.8%, 55.1%, and 69.2%, respectively. Univariate analysis for predictors of dropout revealed a significantly lower risk for patients treated with TACE or RFA prior to OLT. The UCSF study suggested further changes in the current allocation scheme for patients with HCC listed for OLT. A lower initial MELD score followed by a greater incremental increase while on list, especially past six months, may be more beneficial given this pattern of disease progression. Several other centers have also documented a positive influence of ablative therapy on dropout while on the waiting list (46, 47).

The impact (if any) of loco-regional therapy prior to transplant on overall survival and cancer recurrence is not clear. Several studies have failed to demonstrate a survival benefit (11, 48, 49). Conversely, the combined experience from UCSF and Columbia University suggests the opposite (50). Of the 85 patients with T2 and T3 tumors who underwent pre-OLT loco-regional therapy, the five-year recurrence-free survival was nearly 94%. For the other 41 patients who did not undergo preoperative ablation, disease-free survival in the same time interval was decreased to 80.6%. This treatment benefit was more pronounced for those with T3 tumors.

Despite these encouraging results, these data should be interpreted with caution. First, this study, like all others, is hampered by the lack of randomization and includes a small number of patients. Second, the mode and timing of ablative therapy are not consistent. Some patients were treated electively at random time points prior to OLT, while others were treated within 24 hours of surgery. Furthermore, 43% of patients were treated by TACE exclusively, while nearly 10% were treated with a combination of TACE plus either RFA or ethanol injection. The authors acknowledged that the lack of a well-defined protocol may lead to selection bias. While reasonable tumor ablation is pathologically well documented (51), the global utility of loco-regional therapy prior to transplant remains to be determined in a randomized trial (52).

RECURRENCE OF HCC AFTER TRANSPLANT

The reemergence of cancer following transplantation remains a formidable problem (6, 7). Reportedly as high as 40% in some centers (53), recurrent HCC is the rate-limiting obstacle to long-term survival (54). With organ allocation currently based on the preoperative stage of the disease, several factors predictive of outcome have been identified. Early observations by Iwatsuki et al. identified lymph node metastasis and vascular invasion as strong predictors (10). Additionally, both micro- and macrovascular invasion portend a worse outcome and correlate with cancer recurrence (55). Tumor size (56), bilobar disease (29), tumor grade (57), and elevated serum alpha-fetoprotein (55) may negatively influence patient survival.

Several groups have documented the patterns and incidence of recurrent HCC (5–7, 53, 54, 58–60) (Table 1). Roayaie and colleagues observed an 18% incidence of tumor recurrence in 311 patients transplanted for cancer (7). Long-term survival was significantly lower in patients with recurrence versus those without (22% vs. 64% at 5 years post-OLT). While the majority of patients with recurrent tumor had vascular invasion, multivariate analysis suggests that the size, differentiation, and presence of bone metastasis negatively impacted survival. Interestingly, the mean time to tumor recurrence was longest in patients with hepatitis C. Overall, factors associated with cancer recurrence also correlated with earlier recurrence and shorter survival.

Figures from the UNOS database for liver transplantation compared over 900 OLT patients with HCC to over 33,000 without HCC (13). Overall, the five-year survival was 48.2% in patients with HCC versus 74.7% in patients without. Survival improved dramatically over time, as

Table 1
Incidence of Recurrent HCC After Transplant

Author	Number of Patients	% Recurrence
Marsh (53)	178	40.0% (71/178)
Regalia (6)	132	15.9% (21/132)
Hemming (54)	112	9.8% (11/112)
Leung (59)	144	15.3% (11/144)
Shimoda (5)	67	16.4% (11/67)
Schlitt (58)	69	56.5% (39/69)
Roayaie (7)	311	18.3% (57/311)
Margarit (60)	103	14.5% (15/133)

patients transplanted between 1987 and 1991 had a five-year survival of 25%. Conversely, those transplanted between 1996 and 2001 had a five-year survival of 61%. Only 75 of 985 patients developed recurrent tumor. However, preoperative staging data and selection criteria were not available. The experience from the University of Pittsburgh reports an extremely high incidence of recurrence (40%) (53). The authors make several important observations. Macrovascular invasion was the single most influential risk factor identified, as all but one patient recurred. Additionally, all patients with positive margins developed recurrent disease within one year of transplant. Of the 71 patients who suffered a recurrence, only 25 patients recurred in the liver and over 90% recurred within two years of transplantation. Our experience at UCLA reveals a 16% recurrence rate in patients with hepatitis C and HCC. Tumor stage and vascular invasion were associated with a poor outcome (5).While the actual incidence of recurrence varies from center to center, it is clear that several tumor-associated factors hold important prognostic significance. Uniformly, tumor size and presence of vascular invasion have emerged as the most clinically significant characteristics. Interestingly, tumor size may actually predict the presence of vascular invasion (61).

Role of Immunosuppression

Repression of immunosurveillance is only partially responsible for recurrent malignancy posttransplant. A growing body of evidence suggests current immunosuppressive agents may promote a variety of oncogenic changes. Cyclosporine (CsA) induces cellular changes, including increased motility and conversion to an invasive phenotype (62). CsA significantly increased the number of pulmonary metastatic deposits in mice for a variety of tumors. Intrahepatic implantation of a hepatoma cell line, followed by liver transplant at postimplant day 16, revealed a significant survival reduction in CsA-treated animals (63). Furthermore, the incidence of pulmonary metastasis and extrapulmonary recurrence were increased in the CsA treatment group. Clinically, Vivarelli and colleagues reported an increase in five-year recurrence-free survival in patients treated with lower cumulative doses of CsA in the first 12 months following OLT (64). Additionally, they documented a higher mean CsA level in patients with cancer recurrence (65).

Sirolimus (RAPA), a bacterial macrolide, possesses both immunosuppressive and antineoplastic properties. Mechanistically, RAPA binds the mammalian target of rapamycin (mTOR), subsequently inhibiting IL-2-mediated lymphoid expansion (66). Guba and colleagues reported that RAPA inhibits metastatic tumor growth and neovascularization in the liver (67). Alternatively, CsA promotes tumor growth and new blood vessel formation. RAPA decreases vascular endothelial growth factor (VEGF) expression and attenuates the response of endothelial cells to VEGF stimulation. Similar antiproliferative effects of RAPA on hepatoma cells have been documented by other groups (68, 69). Importantly, drug levels at which RAPA promotes antiangiogenic properties are compatible with those used clinically (70).

The first prospective series of patients with HCC treated with sirolimus was recently reported (71). With a protocol designed to wean steroids and calcineurin-inhibitors early postoperatively, they sought to achieve maintenance monotherapy with sirolimus within six months of transplant. Of 40 patients, 19 met the Milan criteria and 21 did not. Cumulatively, four tumor recurrences were observed in the "extended criteria" group and only one in the Milan group. Disease-free survival was not different between the two groups. They concluded that the Milan criteria can be safely extended without compromising patient outcome, and sirolimus monotherapy may have a beneficial effect on recurrence and overall survival. Unfortunately, this series did not include a control group against which to compare the sirolimus protocol. They suggest sirolimus monotherapy may be beneficial by comparing tumor recurrence and postrecurrence survival in this series to that of another center (22). Interestingly, only 25 of 35 surviving patients were maintained on sirolimus monotherapy. Clearly, preclinical data suggest that currently utilized regimens of immunosuppression have a questionable degree of oncologic influence. Whether these actions have a clinically significant impact on tumor recurrence after transplant is not clear.

Surgical Strategy for Recurrent HCC

Few treatment options are available for patients with recurrent cancer after transplantation. Unfortunately, most present with multifocal and/or extrahepatic disease and are not candidates for loco-regional therapy (72). However, for a subgroup of patients, aggressive surgical intervention has recently been advocated. Three groups have reported their results in a small number of patients. A series from Milan included 132 patients transplanted for HCC at three Italian hospitals (6). Overall, 15.9% developed a recurrence at an average of 7.8 months after OLT. Approximately 40% of patients had multiple organ involvement. Seven patients underwent surgical resection for recurrence in the liver, lungs, bone, and skin. Four-year survival was 57%. Survival at the same time interval for unresectable patients was only 14%.

A similar experience from Schlitt and colleagues documented 11 patients with recurrence treated surgically (58). Seven of these 11 patients were alive, with a follow-up of 4.3 years. A report from Mount Sinai Medical Center chronicled 57 recurrences in over 300 patients transplanted for HCC (7). Twelve of the 57 recurrences were treated by either liver or lung resection. Survival at five years was significantly better in patients treated by resection compared to those who were not (47% vs. 10%). While surgical resection for recurrent tumor appears to be a viable treatment option for a subset of patients with cancer recurrence, several challenges remain. The international experience thus far is extremely small. Whether this radical treatment strategy actually confers a long-term survival benefit needs to be confirmed on a larger scale. Further, the number of patients who are actually candidates for post-OLT resection is limited.

LIVER RESECTION AS A "BRIDGE" TO TRANSPLANTATION

The appropriate treatment strategy for patients with good liver function and small cancers has not been well defined (73). Several studies have demonstrated reasonable survival in Childs A patients treated by OLT (74–76). Alternatively, several authors have concluded that overall and disease-free survival are similar after liver resection versus OLT (77–79). With a critical shortage of cadaveric organs, and extended time on the waiting list, some authors have proposed liver resection as first-line therapy in patients with good liver function (80). A product of this debate is the treatment strategy termed "salvage transplantation" (81). As such, primary hepatic resection followed by OLT for HCC recurrence or liver failure has been employed by several centers. Belghiti and colleagues reported a series of 107 patients (82) (Table 2). Seventy patients underwent primary OLT, with 18 patients treated with primary resection. Eleven of these 18 patients underwent "salvage" OLT for cancer recurrence. Both three- and five-year survival between primary and secondary OLT groups were similar.

Margarit and colleagues observed an increased recurrence rate following liver resection for single lesions less than 5 cm in Childs A patients (83). In this series, 59% of patients undergoing resection developed a recurrence, the majority of which were predominantly intrahepatic. The recurrence rate after primary OLT was only 11% and was extrahepatic in 75% of patients. The lungs, adrenal glands, and bones were the most frequent sites of metastasis, which appeared at a mean of 16 months postoperatively. Interestingly, five patients were treated

Table 2
Secondary OLT Following Curative Hepatectomy

Author	Number of Patients	Salvage OLT for HCC Recurrence	Comments
Resection as a "Bridge" to OLT			
Margarit (83)	LR = 37OLT = 36	6	Five-year survival comparable between POLT and SOLT (63% vs. 80%)
Belghiti (82)	LR = 18 OLT = 70	11	Five-year survival comparable between POLT and SOLT (59% vs. 61%)
Poon (80)	LR = 135	2	79% of patients with HCC recurrence after resection eligible for SOLT
Adam (84)	LR = 163 OLT = 195	17	Five-year survival significantly worse for SOLT compared to POLT (29% vs. 58%)

OLT = orthotopic liver transplant; POLT = primary liver transplant; SOLT = salvage liver transplant; LR = liver resection; HCC = hepatocellular carcinoma.

with "salvage OLT" following postresection recurrence with comparable one- and five-year survival to primary OLT. Margarit and colleagues concluded that liver resection may serve as a "bridge" to transplantation in a select group of patients with small tumors and well-compensated disease. Importantly, previous resection did not appear to jeopardize the outcome of subsequent transplantation.

One of the largest experiences with secondary salvage OLT reported conflicting results (84). Seventeen patients underwent secondary OLT after liver resection compared to 195 patients undergoing primary OLT. These authors made several important observations. Of the 69 recurrences after resection, only 17 (25%) were eligible for transplant. Fifty-four percent of patients receiving a salvage OLT suffered a cancer recurrence, the majority of which were intrahepatic. Patients undergoing hepatic resection had a higher operative mortality and blood requirement. Finally, the five-year disease-free survival for salvage and primary OLT was 18% and 58%, respectively. Based on these findings, they advocated that patients at high risk for HCC recurrence (i.e., multiple tumors, presence of vascular invasion) be excluded from a two-stage treatment strategy.

REFERENCES

1. El-Serag HB, Mason AC. Rising incidence of hepatocellular carcinoma in the United States. *N Engl J Med* 1999; 340:745–50.
2. Wong JB, McQuillan GM, McHutchison JG, Poynard T. Estimating future hepatitis C morbidity, mortality, and costs in the United States. *Am J Public Health* 2000; 90:1562–9.
3. Everson GT. Increasing incidence and pretransplantation screening of hepatocellular carcinoma. *Liver Transpl* 2000; 6:S2–S10.
4. Llovet JM, Schwartz M, Mazzaferro V. Resection and liver transplantation for hepatocellular carcinoma. *Semin Liver Dis* 2005; 25:181–200.
5. Shimoda M, Ghobrial RM, Carmody IC, Anselmo DM, Farmer DG, Yersiz H, Chen P, et al. Predictors of survival after liver transplantation for hepatocellular carcinoma associated with hepatitis C. *Liver Transpl* 2004; 10:1478–86.
6. Regalia E, Fassati LR, Valente U, Pulvirenti A, Damilano I, Dardano G, Montalto F, et al. Pattern and management of recurrent hepatocellular carcinoma after liver transplantation. *J Hepatobil Pancr Surg* 1998; 5:29–34.
7. Roayaie S, Schwartz JD, Sung MW, Emre SH, Miller CM, Gondolesi GE, Krieger NR, et al. Recurrence of hepatocellular carcinoma after liver transplant: Patterns and prognosis. *Liver Transpl* 2004; 10:534–40.
8. Sharma P, Balan V, Hernandez JL, Harper AM, Edwards EB, Rodriguez-Luna H, Byrne T, et al. Liver transplantation for hepatocellular carcinoma: The MELD impact. *Liver Transpl* 2004; 10:36–41.
9. Yao FY, Roberts JP. Applying expanded criteria to liver transplantation for hepatocellular carcinoma: Too much too soon, or is now the time? *Liver Transpl* 2004; 10:919–21.
10. Iwatsuki S, Starzl TE, Sheahan DG, Yokoyama I, Demetris AJ, Todo S, Tzakis AG, et al. Hepatic resection versus transplantation for hepatocellular carcinoma. *Ann Surg* 1991; 214:221–8; disc 228–9.
11. Mazzaferro V, Regalia E, Doci R, Andreola S, Pulvirenti A, Bozzetti F, Montalto F, et al. Liver transplantation for the treatment of small hepatocellular carcinomas in patients with cirrhosis. *N Engl J Med* 1996; 334:693–9.
12. Broelsch CE, Frilling A, Malago M. Should we expand the criteria for liver transplantation for hepatocellular carcinoma?—Yes, of course! *J Hepatol* 2005; 43:569–73.
13. Yoo HY, Patt CH, Geschwind JF, Thuluvath PJ. The outcome of liver transplantation in patients with hepatocellular carcinoma in the United States between 1988 and 2001: Five-year survival has improved significantly with time. *J Clin Oncol* 2003; 21:4329–35.

14. Pokorny H, Gnant M, Rasoul-Rockenschaub S, Gollackner B, Steiner B, Steger G, Steininger R, et al. Does additional doxorubicin chemotherapy improve outcome in patients with hepatocellular carcinoma treated by liver transplantation? *Am J Transpl* 2005; 5:788–94.

15. Marsh JW, Dvorchik I. Liver organ allocation for hepatocellular carcinoma: Are we sure? *Liver Transpl* 2003; 9:693–6.

16. Olthoff KM, Millis JM, Rosove MH, Goldstein LI, Ramming KP, Busuttil RW. Is liver transplantation justified for the treatment of hepatic malignancies? *Arch Surg* 1990; 125:1261–6; disc 1266–8.

17. Figueras J, Jaurrieta E, Valls C, Benasco C, Rafecas A, Xiol X, Fabregat J, et al. Survival after liver transplantation in cirrhotic patients with and without hepatocellular carcinoma: A comparative study. *Hepatology* 1997; 25:1485–9.

18. Llovet JM, Bruix J, Fuster J, Castells A, Garcia-Valdecasas JC, Grande L, Franca A, et al. Liver transplantation for small hepatocellular carcinoma: The tumor-node-metastasis classification does not have prognostic power. *Hepatology* 1998; 27:1572–7.

19. Herrero JI, Sangro B, Quiroga J, Pardo F, Herraiz M, Cienfuegos JA, Prieto J. Influence of tumor characteristics on the outcome of liver transplantation among patients with liver cirrhosis and hepatocellular carcinoma. *Liver Transpl* 2001; 7:631–6.

20. Iwatsuki S, Dvorchik I, Marsh JW, Madariaga JR, Carr B, Fung JJ, Starzl TE. Liver transplantation for hepatocellular carcinoma: A proposal of a prognostic scoring system. *J Am Coll Surg* 2000; 191:389–94.

21. Yao FY, Ferrell L, Bass NM, Watson JJ, Bacchetti P, Venook A, Ascher NL, et al. Liver transplantation for hepatocellular carcinoma: Expansion of the tumor size limits does not adversely impact survival. *Hepatology* 2001; 33:1394–403.

22. Yao FY, Ferrell L, Bass NM, Bacchetti P, Ascher NL, Roberts JP. Liver transplantation for hepatocellular carcinoma: Comparison of the proposed UCSF criteria with the Milan criteria and the Pittsburgh modified TNM criteria. *Liver Transpl* 2002; 8:765–74.

23. Hiatt JR, Carmody IC, Busuttil RW. Should we expand the criteria for hepatocellular carcinoma with living-donor liver transplantation?—No, never. *J Hepatol* 2005; 43:573–7.

24. Liu C, Frilling A, Sotiropoulos GC, Weber F, Nadalin S, Malago M, Broelsch CE. Living donor liver transplantation for recurrent hepatocellular carcinoma. *Transpl Int* 2005; 18:889.

25. Wachs ME, Bak TE, Karrer FM, Everson GT, Shrestha R, Trouillot TE, Mandell MS, et al. Adult living donor liver transplantation using a right hepatic lobe. *Transplantation* 1998; 66:1313–6.

26. Trotter JF, Wachs M, Everson GT, Kam I. Adult-to-adult transplantation of the right hepatic lobe from a living donor. *N Engl J Med* 2002; 346:1074–82.

27. Olthoff KM, Merion RM, Ghobrial RM, Abecassis MM, Fair JH, Fisher RA, Freise CE, et al. Outcomes of 385 adult-to-adult living donor liver transplant recipients: A report from the A2ALL Consortium. *Ann Surg* 2005; 242:314–23.

28. Lo CM, Fan ST, Liu CL, Chan SC, Wong J. The role and limitation of living donor liver transplantation for hepatocellular carcinoma. *Liver Transpl* 2004; 10:440–7.

29. Todo S, Furukawa H. Living donor liver transplantation for adult patients with hepatocellular carcinoma: Experience in Japan. *Ann Surg* 2004; 240:451–9.

30. Hwang S, Lee SG, Joh JW, Suh KS, Kim DG. Liver transplantation for adult patients with hepatocellular carcinoma in Korea: Comparison between cadaveric donor and living donor liver transplantations. *Liver Transpl* 2005; 11:1265–72.

31. Busuttil RW, Tanaka K. The utility of marginal donors in liver transplantation. *Liver Transpl* 2003; 9:651–63.

32. Seu P, Imagawa DK, Olthoff KM, Yersiz H, Rosenthal TJ, Sellers CA, Ginther G, et al. A prospective study on the reliability and cost effectiveness of preoperative ultrasound screening of the "marginal" liver donor. *Transplantation* 1996; 62:129–30.

33. Alexander JW, Vaughn WK. The use of "marginal" donors for organ transplantation. The influence of donor age on outcome. *Transplantation* 1991; 51:135–41.

34. Mor E, Klintmalm GB, Gonwa TA, Solomon H, Holman MJ, Gibbs JF, Watemberg I, et al. The use of marginal donors for liver transplantation. A retrospective study of 365 liver donors. *Transplantation* 1992; 53:383–6.

35. De Carlis L, Sansalone CV, Rondinara GF, Colella G, Slim AO, Rossetti O, Aseni P, et al. Is the use of marginal donors justified in liver transplantation? Analysis of results and proposal of modern criteria. *Transpl Int* 1996; 9(Suppl 1):S414–S417.

36. Rocha MB, Boin IF, Escanhoela CA, Leonardi LS. Can the use of marginal liver donors change recipient survival rate? *Transpl Proc* 2004; 36:914–5.

37. Montalti R, Nardo B, Bertelli R, Beltempo P, Puviani L, Vivarelli M, Cavallari A. Donor pool expansion in liver transplantation. *Transpl Proc* 2004; 36:520–2.

38. Tisone G, Manzia TM, Zazza S, De Liguori Carino N, Ciceroni C, De Luca I, Toti L, et al. Marginal donors in liver transplantation. *Transpl Proc* 2004; 36:525–6.

39. Nardo B, Masetti M, Urbani L, Caraceni P, Montalti R, Filipponi F, Mosca F, et al. Liver transplantation from donors aged 80 years and over: Pushing the limit. *Am J Transpl* 2004; 4:1139–47.

40. Sotiropoulos GC, Malago M, Molmenti E, Paul A, Nadalin S, Brokalaki E, Kuhl H, et al. Liver transplantation for hepatocellular carcinoma in cirrhosis: Is clinical tumor classification before transplantation realistic? *Transplantation* 2005; 79:483–7.

41. Vogl TJ, Hanninen EL, Bechstein WO, Neuhaus P, Schumacher G, Felix R. Biphasic spiral computed tomography versus digital subtraction angiography for evaluation of arterial thrombosis after orthotopic liver transplantation. *Invest Radiol* 1998; 33:136–40.

42. Libbrecht L, Bielen D, Verslype C, Vanbeckevoort D, Pirenne J, Nevens F, Desmet V, et al. Focal lesions in cirrhotic explant livers: Pathological evaluation and accuracy of pretransplantation imaging examinations. *Liver Transpl* 2002; 8:749–61.

43. Krinsky GA, Lee VS, Theise ND, Weinreb JC, Morgan GR, Diflo T, John D, et al. Transplantation for hepatocellular carcinoma and cirrhosis: Sensitivity of magnetic resonance imaging. *Liver Transpl* 2002; 8:1156–64.

44. Kaihara S, Kiuchi T, Ueda M, Oike F, Fujimoto Y, Ogawa K, Kozaki K, et al. Living-donor liver transplantation for hepatocellular carcinoma. *Transplantation* 2003; 75:S37–S40.

45. Yao FY, Bass NM, Nikolai B, Merriman R, Davern TJ, Kerlan R, Ascher NL, et al. A follow-up analysis of the pattern and predictors of dropout from the waiting list

for liver transplantation in patients with hepatocellular carcinoma: Implications for the current organ allocation policy. *Liver Transpl* 2003; 9:684–92.

46. Graziadei IW, Sandmueller H, Waldenberger P, Koenigsrainer A, Nachbaur K, Jaschke W, Margreiter R, et al. Chemoembolization followed by liver transplantation for hepatocellular carcinoma impedes tumor progression while on the waiting list and leads to excellent outcome. *Liver Transpl* 2003; 9:557–63.

47. Llovet JM, Mas X, Aponte JJ, Fuster J, Navasa M, Christensen E, Rodes J, et al. Cost effectiveness of adjuvant therapy for hepatocellular carcinoma during the waiting list for liver transplantation. *Gut* 2002; 50:123–8.

48. Oldhafer KJ, Chavan A, Fruhauf NR, Flemming P, Schlitt HJ, Kubicka S, Nashan B, et al. Arterial chemoembolization before liver transplantation in patients with hepatocellular carcinoma: Marked tumor necrosis, but no survival benefit? *J Hepatol* 1998; 29:953–9.

49. Decaens T, Roudot-Thoraval F, Bresson-Hadni S, Meyer C, Gugenheim J, Durand F, Bernard PH, et al. Impact of pretransplantation transarterial chemoembolization on survival and recurrence after liver transplantation for hepatocellular carcinoma. *Liver Transpl* 2005; 11:767–75.

50. Yao FY, Kinkhabwala M, LaBerge JM, Bass NM, Brown R, Jr., Kerlan R, Venook A, et al. The impact of pre-operative loco-regional therapy on outcome after liver transplantation for hepatocellular carcinoma. *Am J Transpl* 2005; 5:795–804.

51. Lu DS, Yu NC, Raman SS, Lassman C, Tong MJ, Britten C, Durazo F, et al. Percutaneous radiofrequency ablation of hepatocellular carcinoma as a bridge to liver transplantation. *Hepatology* 2005; 41:1130–7.

52. Palmer DH, Johnson PJ. Pre-operative locoregional therapy and liver transplantation for hepatocellular carcinoma: Time for a randomized controlled trial. *Am J Transpl* 2005; 5:641–2.

53. Marsh JW, Dvorchik I, Subotin M, Balan V, Rakela J, Popechitelev EP, Subbotin V, et al. The prediction of risk of recurrence and time to recurrence of hepatocellular carcinoma after orthotopic liver transplantation: A pilot study. *Hepatology* 1997; 26:444–50.

54. Hemming AW, Cattral MS, Reed AI, Van Der Werf WJ, Greig PD, Howard RJ. Liver transplantation for hepatocellular carcinoma. *Ann Surg* 2001; 233:652–9.

55. Shetty K, Timmins K, Brensinger C, Furth EE, Rattan S, Sun W, Rosen M, et al. Liver transplantation for hepatocellular carcinoma: Validation of present selection criteria in predicting outcome. *Liver Transpl* 2004; 10:911–8.

56. Lohe F, Angele MK, Gerbes AL, Lohrs U, Jauch KW, Schauer RJ. Tumour size is an important predictor for the outcome after liver transplantation for hepatocellular carcinoma. *Eur J Surg Oncol* 2005; 31:994–9.

57. Jonas S, Bechstein WO, Steinmuller T, Herrmann M, Radke C, Berg T, Settmacher U, et al. Vascular invasion and histopathologic grading determine outcome after liver transplantation for hepatocellular carcinoma in cirrhosis. *Hepatology* 2001; 33:1080–6.

58. Schlitt HJ, Neipp M, Weimann A, Oldhafer KJ, Schmoll E, Boeker K, Nashan B, et al. Recurrence patterns of hepatocellular and fibrolamellar carcinoma after liver transplantation. *J Clin Oncol* 1999; 17:324–31.

59. Leung JY, Zhu AX, Gordon FD, Pratt DS, Mithoefer A, Garrigan K, Terella A, et al. Liver transplantation outcomes for early-stage hepatocellular carcinoma: Results of a multicenter study. *Liver Transpl* 2004; 10:1343–54.
60. Margarit C, Charco R, Hidalgo E, Allende H, Castells L, Bilbao I. Liver transplantation for malignant diseases: Selection and pattern of recurrence. *World J Surg* 2002; 26:257–63.
61. Pawlik TM, Delman KA, Vauthey JN, Nagorney DM, Ng IO, Ikai I, Yamaoka Y, et al. Tumor size predicts vascular invasion and histologic grade: Implications for selection of surgical treatment for hepatocellular carcinoma. *Liver Transpl* 2005; 11:1086–92.
62. Hojo M, Morimoto T, Maluccio M, Asano T, Morimoto K, Lagman M, Shimbo T, et al. Cyclosporine induces cancer progression by a cell-autonomous mechanism. *Nature* 1999; 397:530–4.
63. Freise CE, Ferrell L, Liu T, Ascher NL, Roberts JP. Effect of systemic cyclosporine on tumor recurrence after liver transplantation in a model of hepatocellular carcinoma. *Transplantation* 1999; 67:510–3.
64. Vivarelli M, Cucchetti A, Piscaglia F, La Barba G, Bolondi L, Cavallari A, Pinna AD. Analysis of risk factors for tumor recurrence after liver transplantation for hepatocellular carcinoma: Key role of immunosuppression. *Liver Transpl* 2005; 11:497–503.
65. Vivarelli M, Bellusci R, Cucchetti A, Cavrini G, De Ruvo N, Aden AA, La Barba G, et al. Low recurrence rate of hepatocellular carcinoma after liver transplantation: Better patient selection or lower immunosuppression? *Transplantation* 2002; 74:1746–51.
66. Wiederrecht GJ, Sabers CJ, Brunn GJ, Martin MM, Dumont FJ, Abraham RT. Mechanism of action of rapamycin: New insights into the regulation of G1-phase progression in eukaryotic cells. *Prog Cell Cycle Res* 1995; 1:53–71.
67. Guba M, von Breitenbuch P, Steinbauer M, Koehl G, Flegel S, Hornung M, Bruns CJ, et al. Rapamycin inhibits primary and metastatic tumor growth by antiangiogenesis: Involvement of vascular endothelial growth factor. *Nat Med* 2002; 8:128–35.
68. Schumacher G, Oidtmann M, Rosewicz S, Langrehr J, Jonas S, Mueller AR, Rueggeberg A, et al. Sirolimus inhibits growth of human hepatoma cells in contrast to tacrolimus, which promotes cell growth. *Transpl Proc* 2002; 34:1392–3.
69. Schumacher G, Oidtmann M, Rueggeberg A, Jacob D, Jonas S, Langrehr JM, Neuhaus R, et al. Sirolimus inhibits growth of human hepatoma cells alone or combined with tacrolimus, while tacrolimus promotes cell growth. *World J Gastroenterol* 2005; 11:1420–5.
70. Guba M, Koehl GE, Neppl E, Doenecke A, Steinbauer M, Schlitt HJ, Jauch KW, et al. Dosing of rapamycin is critical to achieve an optimal antiangiogenic effect against cancer. *Transpl Int* 2005; 18:89–94.
71. Kneteman NM, Oberholzer J, Al Saghier M, Meeberg GA, Blitz M, Ma MM, Wong WW, et al. Sirolimus-based immunosuppression for liver transplantation in the presence of extended criteria for hepatocellular carcinoma. *Liver Transpl* 2004; 10:1301–11.
72. Schwartz M, Konstadoulakis M, Roayaie S. Recurrence of hepatocellular carcinoma after liver transplantation: Is immunosuppression a factor? *Liver Transpl* 2005; 11:494–6.

73. Llovet JM, Bruix J, Gores GJ. Surgical resection versus transplantation for early hepatocellular carcinoma: Clues for the best strategy. *Hepatology* 2000; 31:1019–21.

74. Michel J, Suc B, Montpeyroux F, Hachemanne S, Blanc P, Domergue J, Mouiel J, et al. Liver resection or transplantation for hepatocellular carcinoma? Retrospective analysis of 215 patients with cirrhosis. *J Hepatol* 1997; 26:1274–80.

75. Figueras J, Jaurrieta E, Valls C, Ramos E, Serrano T, Rafecas A, Fabregat J, et al. Resection or transplantation for hepatocellular carcinoma in cirrhotic patients: Outcomes based on indicated treatment strategy. *J Am Coll Surg* 2000; 190:580–7.

76. Sarasin FP, Giostra E, Mentha G, Hadengue A. Partial hepatectomy or orthotopic liver transplantation for the treatment of resectable hepatocellular carcinoma? A cost-effectiveness perspective. *Hepatology* 1998; 28:436–42.

77. Otto G, Heuschen U, Hofmann WJ, Krumm G, Hinz U, Herfarth C. Survival and recurrence after liver transplantation versus liver resection for hepatocellular carcinoma: A retrospective analysis. *Ann Surg* 1998; 227:424–32.

78. Pichlmayr R, Weimann A, Oldhafer KJ, Schlitt HJ, Tusch G, Raab R. Appraisal of transplantation for malignant tumours of the liver with special reference to early stage hepatocellular carcinoma. *Eur J Surg Oncol* 1998; 24:60–7.

79. Yamamoto J, Iwatsuki S, Kosuge T, Dvorchik I, Shimada K, Marsh JW, Yamasaki S, et al. Should hepatomas be treated with hepatic resection or transplantation? *Cancer* 1999; 86:1151–8.

80. Poon RT, Fan ST, Lo CM, Liu CL, Wong J. Long-term survival and pattern of recurrence after resection of small hepatocellular carcinoma in patients with preserved liver function: Implications for a strategy of salvage transplantation. *Ann Surg* 2002; 235:373–82.

81. Bismuth H, Majno PE, Adam R. Liver transplantation for hepatocellular carcinoma. *Semin Liver Dis* 1999; 19:311–22.

82. Belghiti J, Cortes A, Abdalla EK, Regimbeau JM, Prakash K, Durand F, Sommacale D, et al. Resection prior to liver transplantation for hepatocellular carcinoma. *Ann Surg* 2003; 238:885–92.

83. Margarit C, Escartin A, Castells L, Vargas V, Allende E, Bilbao I. Resection for hepatocellular carcinoma is a good option in Child–Turcotte–Pugh class A patients with cirrhosis who are eligible for liver transplantation. *Liver Transpl* 2005; 11:1242–51.

84. Adam R, Azoulay D, Castaing D, Eshkenazy R, Pascal G, Hashizume K, Samuel D, et al. Liver resection as a bridge to transplantation for hepatocellular carcinoma on cirrhosis: A reasonable strategy? *Ann Surg* 2003; 238:508–18.

7 Liver Transplantation and the Hepatopulmonary Syndrome

David T. Palma, MD
and Michael B. Fallon, MD

Abstract

The hepatopulmonary syndrome (HPS) occurs in as many as 15–20% of patients with cirrhosis; mortality is significantly increased compared to cirrhotic patients without HPS. The only proven effective therapy for HPS is orthotopic liver transplantation (OLT), which should be considered when severe hypoxemia is present. The natural history of HPS without liver transplantation is dismal. While post-OLT mortality is increased in patients with HPS relative to that reported in non-HPS patients, overall outcomes are favorable in properly selected patients. The higher mortality associated with HPS has led to the policy of increasing priority for OLT in selected HPS patients through a Model for End-Stage Liver Disease (MELD) score

From: *Clinical Gastroenterology: Liver Transplantation: Challenging Controversies and Topics*
Edited by: G. T. Everson and J. F. Trotter, DOI: 10.1007/978-1-60327-028-1_7,
© Humana Press, Totowa, NJ

exception. There is currently no established protocol to screen for HPS in OLT candidates. However, a resting PaO_2 < 65–60 mmHg identifies patients who qualify, or who may sufficiently deteriorate over a short time frame to qualify, for MELD exception criteria. In patients with HPS awaiting OLT, no specific therapies are available to improve intrapulmonary vasodilatation. The perioperative management of HPS patients presents particular clinical challenges.

Key Words: Hepatopulmonary syndrome; Hypoxia; Intrapulmonary shunt; Pulmonary disease

BACKGROUND

The hepatopulmonary syndrome (HPS) occurs when pulmonary microvascular dilatation impairs arterial oxygenation in the setting of liver disease or portal hypertension (1). The syndrome is recognized in as many as 15–20% of patients with cirrhosis (2), and mortality is significantly increased in such patients relative to cirrhotic patients without HPS (3, 4). Orthotopic liver transplantation (OLT) is currently the only proven effective therapy for HPS and should be considered when severe hypoxemia is present (1, 3, 4).

This chapter will review the significance of HPS in OLT, provide guidelines for the diagnosis and screening of OLT candidates for HPS, and address salient issues related to transplant candidacy and management.

SIGNIFICANCE OF HPS IN OLT

Outcome of HPS Without OLT

The natural history of hepatopulmonary syndrome is incompletely characterized. Most patients appear to develop progressive intrapulmonary vasodilatation and worsening gas exchange over time (3, 5), and spontaneous improvement is rare (6). To date, two single-center studies have accounted for the majority of available data concerning the natural history and prognosis of HPS (3, 4).

In one prospective study, 111 patients with cirrhosis were evaluated, 20 of whom had HPS. The median survival was 4.8 and 35.3 months for patients with HPS and those without HPS who did not undergo OLT, respectively [Fig. 1(a)] (4). Mortality remained higher in those with HPS after adjusting for the severity of liver disease. In patients with HPS, mortality largely resulted from complications of liver disease or portal hypertension, and it correlated with the degree of hypoxemia (4).

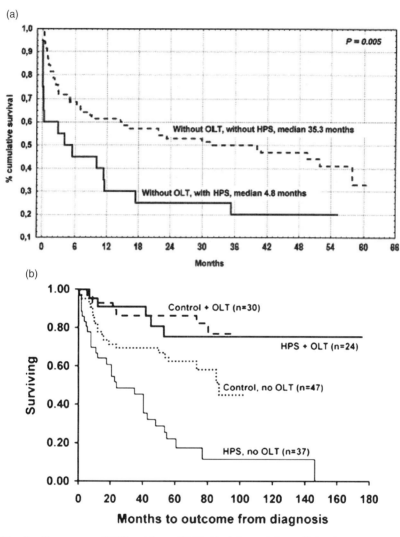

Fig. 1. Outcome of HPS without OLT. (a) Adapted from Schenk et al., *Gastroenterology* 2003; 125:1042–52. (b) Adapted from Swanson et al., *Hepatology* 2005; 41:1122–9.

Another recent retrospective study examined 61 patients with cirrhosis and HPS, 37 of whom did not undergo OLT. Patients with HPS who did not undergo OLT had a median survival of 24 months and a five-year survival of 23%. In contrast, those without HPS who did not undergo OLT ($n = 47$) had a median survival of 87 months and a five-year survival of 63% [Fig. 1(b)] (3). However, a subset of the HPS group not undergoing OLT were excluded from surgery due to comorbidities that may have influenced survival.

Together, these data support that mortality in patients with cirrhosis not undergoing OLT is significantly increased in those with HPS relative to those without HPS and that the degree of hypoxemia and severity of hepatic dysfunction adversely influence outcome (3, 4). Future investigation is needed to precisely characterize the natural history of HPS and to define specific factors that influence mortality and OLT candidacy in these patients.

Outcome of HPS with OLT

Over the last two decades, opinions and policies concerning OLT in patients with HPS have evolved considerably. Until the late 1980s, many investigators and transplant centers regarded the hypoxemia of HPS to be irreversible and therefore a contraindication to OLT (7, 8). This was based on several cases in which hypoxemia in patients with HPS persisted following OLT. Since that time, there has been substantial evidence to support that OLT is an effective therapy for HPS, resulting in complete resolution or significant improvement in gas exchange in over 85% of patients (9). However, the length of time to normalization of arterial hypoxemia post-OLT is variable and may be more than one year (10).

In addition to the delayed resolution of HPS after OLT, postoperative mortality has also been found to be increased in patients with HPS. A single prospective study has assessed the severity of HPS as a predictor of post-OLT outcome in a cohort of 24 patients with HPS (overall mortality 29%) (11). Post-OLT mortality was significantly higher in severe HPS and was in part attributable to the development of unusual postoperative complications recognized in HPS patients (pulmonary hypertension, cerebral embolic hemorrhages, and immediate postoperative deoxygenation requiring prolonged mechanical ventilation) (12–16). The strongest predictor of mortality was a preoperative $PaO_2 \leq 50\,mmHg$ alone or in combination with a macroaggregated albumin shunt fraction $\geq 20\%$ (11). Two smaller prospective studies and three retrospective studies have also found increased postoperative mortality in HPS patients ranging from 21–50% (Table 1). Collectively, these studies support that post-OLT mortality is increased in patients with HPS relative to that reported in non-HPS patients. The severity of preoperative hypoxemia and underlying liver disease appear to be factors that increase mortality.

Table 1
Outcome of HPS with OLT

	Type	No. of HPS	Post-op Mortality (%)	Pre-op PaO$_2$ (mmHg)	Ref.
Taille	Retrospective	23	30	51.4 (33–64)	(3)
Arguedas	Prospective	24	29	43 (35–51)	(4)
Swanson	Retrospective	24	21	40.6 (33–51)	(11)
Schenk	Prospective	7	42	66 (60–79)	(17)
Collison	Retrospective	6	50	57.2 (40–84)	(18)
Schiffer	Prospective	9	33	60 (52–70)	(19)
Total		93	34		

MELD EXCEPTION

The observation that HPS increases mortality and that post-OLT outcome worsens in cases of advanced HPS has led to the policy in U.S. centers of increasing priority for OLT in patients with HPS and significant hypoxemia (20). While significant data are available to support additional priority for patients with HPS (3, 4), a preliminary report utilizing the UNOS database has not found increased waitlist mortality in patients receiving MELD exception for HPS relative to all others (21). However, it is important to recognize that the current UNOS database does not contain information on cardiopulmonary parameters, causes of death, or relationships between outcome and oxygenation. In addition, no uniform HPS screening protocol is used across transplant centers. These factors limit interpretation of the UNOS data and emphasize the need to collect and interpret more complete information regarding MELD exception for HPS.

Other areas of uncertainty concerning the current MELD exception for HPS include how oxygenation changes over time and how other factors influence mortality in HPS. In one small HPS cohort, PaO$_2$ declined in 12 of the 14 (85%) patients over time, with an average decline of 5 mmHg per year (3). No studies have addressed whether specific complications of cirrhosis (bleeding, SBP, etc.) or rapid changes in hepatic synthetic function influence oxygenation in cirrhotic patients with HPS. Therefore, more information on how oxygenation changes and on factors that influence HPS progression and outcome is needed to optimize allocation of MELD exception points and post-OLT survival.

DIAGNOSIS AND SCREENING

The diagnosis of HPS is defined by the presence of abnormal arterial gas exchange on room air due to intrapulmonary vascular dilatation in the setting of liver disease or portal hypertension (1). The prevalence of HPS varies based on whether gas exchange abnormalities are defined by a widened alveolar-arterial oxygen gradient ($AaPO_2$) or arterial hypoxemia (PaO_2) and ranges from 12–32% (11, 22–26). From a practical standpoint, in the setting of OLT evaluation, detecting all HPS patients with a resting $PaO_2 < 60$–65 mmHg is a reasonable standard to identify patients who qualify or may sufficiently deteriorate over a short time frame to qualify for MELD exception criteria.

There is currently no established protocol to screen for HPS in OLT candidates. Clinical features such as orthodeoxia and clubbing, although commonly present in HPS, are insensitive for screening. In addition, there is variability in routine screening for cardiopulmonary disease among OLT centers. Finally, the spectrum of oxygenation abnormalities in HPS ranges from mild increases in the alveolar-arterial oxygen gradient to profound hypoxemia, and the target group for detection with screening during OLT evaluation is not clearly defined.

One practical approach to identifying clinically important HPS in OLT candidates is to screen all patients with pulse oximetry to detect hypoxemia and contrast echocardiography to detect intrapulmonary vasodilatation (Fig. 2). In one large prospective study of 200 OLT candidates, pulse oximetry was an effective technique to screen for

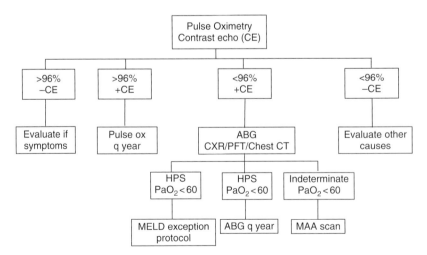

Fig. 2. HPS screening in OLT candidates.

hypoxemia in patients with cirrhosis (25). Using a screening oximetry threshold of 96% or less to trigger obtaining an arterial blood gas (ABG) would have detected all patients with a $PaO_2 < 60$ mmHg and resulted in ABG testing in only 14% of the cohort. Microbubble transthoracic contrast echocardiography (CE), the most sensitive test to detect intra-pulmonary vasodilatation (26), is then performed. Although qualitative, this test also screens for pulmonary hypertension and frequently distin-guishes intracardiac and intrapulmonary shunting (26)

Using a combination of these two tests, patients may be stratified rel-ative to the presence of HPS and the need for further work-up (Fig. 2). If oximetry reveals a value higher than 96% and CE shows no intra-pulmonary vasodilatation, then HPS is not present and patients may be reevaluated in the future if symptoms develop. If oximetry exceeds 96% and CE shows intrapulmonary vasodilatation, then pulse oximetry surveillance yearly to detect the development of hypoxemia is under-taken. If oximetry is less than 96% and CE shows intrapulmonary va-sodilatation, then clinically significant HPS is likely and further testing is indicated to exclude intrinsic cardiopulmonary disease, assess for sig-nificant ascites or hepatic hydrothorax, and define the severity of HPS. If further testing is negative and the PaO_2 is under 60 mmHg, then HPS of sufficient severity to consider MELD exception is present. If HPS is less severe ($PaO_2 > 60$ mmHg), then interval ABG determinations to assess for progression are reasonable. If significant intrinsic cardiopul-monary disease or fluid retention, hypoxemia, and a positive CE are present, then the severity of HPS may be difficult to gauge. In this setting, radionuclide scanning with Tc99m-macroaggregated albumin (MAA) may be useful in defining the contribution of HPS to abnormal gas exchange (27). If the MAA reveals increased shunting ($>6\%$), HPS is likely an important contributor to hypoxemia (27). If oximetry is less than 96% and intrapulmonary vasodilatation is absent, then evaluation for other causes of hypoxemia is appropriate.

TRANSPLANT CANDIDACY AND MANAGEMENT

There are currently no proven medical therapies for HPS. There-fore, all patients with HPS who are otherwise suitable candidates should be considered for OLT. In severely hypoxemic patients ($PaO_2 < 60$ mmHg), assignment of MELD exception points is an appropri-ate consideration to facilitate OLT and improve outcome. Post-OLT mortality appears to be highest (approximately 60%) in HPS patients with profound hypoxemia ($PaO_2 < 50$ mmHg) (11). There are presently insufficient data to definitively establish a severity of HPS where OLT should not be undertaken. However, when considering patients with profound HPS for OLT, the presence of comorbidities should be considered because they may adversely influence outcome during the often prolonged recovery phase following OLT. In addition, patients with severe HPS who also have a minimal response to 100% oxygen testing (PaO_2 < 100 mmHg) might be expected to have particular difficulty with oxygenation during the postoperative period. Expanded prospective studies are needed to characterize the factors that influence post-OLT outcomes in patients with severe HPS.

In patients with HPS awaiting OLT, no specific therapies are available to improve intrapulmonary vasodilatation. One small study suggests that garlic may improve oxygenation in a subset of patients (28), and a case report suggests that antibiotics targeted at intestinal decontamination and bacterial translocation may be beneficial (29). The latter concept has support in animal models (30). In all patients with significant oxygenation abnormalities (PaO_2 < 60 mmHg or pulse oximetry < 95%) at rest or with exertion, the administration of supplemental oxygen is appropriate, based on the concept that the presence of hypoxemia itself may contribute to mortality in HPS (4).

In patients with HPS who have undergone OLT, the perioperative period may present particular clinical challenges. Worsening hypoxemia may occur in the early postoperative period and should be anticipated. Innovative approaches such as frequent body positioning (31) or inhaled NO (32, 33) may be useful in improving gas exchange during this period. Since many patients with severe HPS who do not recover have prolonged intensive care unit stays and unique postoperative complications (12–16), meticulous critical care, with particular attention to preventing infection, is an important goal. In our experience, two additional clinical considerations frequently arise in patients with severe hypoxemia in the early postoperative period. The first is the continued use of aggressive diuresis to treat hypoxemia due to HPS after having accounted for perioperative fluid accumulation and shifts. In this situation, prerenal azotemia and thickened respiratory secretions with the development of mucus plugging have occurred and may prolong time in the intensive care unit. The second is the continuation of mechanical ventilation for hypoxemia due to persistent intrapulmonary vasodilatation in patients otherwise recovering well from OLT. In these patients, extubation and administration of maximal oxygen concentrations may decrease complications related to prolonged ventilation and the need for management within an intensive care unit.

SUMMARY

HPS is recognized in as many as 15–20% of patients with cirrhosis, and mortality is significantly increased in such patients relative to cirrhotic patients without HPS. OLT is currently the only effective therapy for HPS, resulting in complete resolution or significant improvement in gas exchange in over 85% of patients. However, resolution of arterial hypoxemia following OLT is often delayed and post-OLT mortality is increased in patients with HPS relative to non-HPS patients. The severity of preoperative hypoxemia and underlying liver disease appear to be factors that increase mortality. In severely hypoxemic patients ($PaO_2 <$ 60 mmHg), the consideration for MELD exception points is appropriate to facilitate OLT and improve outcome. However, more information on how oxygenation changes and on factors that influence HPS progression and outcome is needed to optimize allocation of MELD exception points and post-OLT survival. Used in combination, pulse oximetry and contrast echocardiography can stratify OLT candidates relative to the presence of HPS and the need for further work-up. In HPS patients who have undergone OLT, worsening of hypoxemia may occur in the early postoperative period and should be anticipated. Since many patients with severe HPS who do not recover have prolonged intensive care unit stays and unique postoperative complications, meticulous critical care, with particular attention to preventing infection, is an important goal.

REFERENCES

1. Rodriguez-Roisin R, Krowka MJ, Herve P, Fallon MB, on behalf of the ERS Task Force Pulmonary-Hepatic Vascular Disorders Scientific Committee ERS Task Force PHD Scientific Committee. Pulmonary-hepatic vascular disorders (PHD). *Eur Respir J* 2004; 24:861–80.
2. Fallon MB, Abrams GA. Pulmonary dysfunction in chronic liver disease. *Hepatology* 2000; 32:859–65.
3. Swanson KL, Wiesner RH, Krowka MJ. Natural history of hepatopulmonary syndrome: Impact of liver transplantation. *Hepatology* 2005; 41:1122–9.
4. Schenk P, Schoniger-Hekele M, Fuhrmann V, Madl C, Silberhumer G, Muller C. Prognostic significance of the hepatopulmonary syndrome in patients with cirrhosis. *Gastroenterology* 2003; 125:1042–52.
5. Krowka MJ, Dickson ER, Cortese DA. Hepatopulmonary syndrome: Clinical observations and lack of therapeutic response to somatostatin analogue. *Chest* 1993; 104:515–21.
6. Saunders KB, Fernando SSD, Dalton HR, Joseph A. Spontaneous improvement in a patient with the hepatopulmonary syndrome assessed by serial exercise tests. *Thorax* 1994; 49:725–7.
7. Herve P, Lebrec D, Brenot F, Simonneau G, Humbert M, Sitbon O, et al. Pulmonary vascular disorders in portal hypertension. *Eur Respir J* 1998; 11:1153–66.

8. Krowka MJ. Hepatopulmonary syndromes. *Gut* 2000; 40:1–4.

9. Lange PA, Stoller JK. The hepatopulmonary syndrome: Effect of liver transplantation. *Clin Chest Med* 1996; 17:115–23.

10. Philit F, Wiesendanger T, Gille D, Boillot O, Cordier JF. Late resolution of hepatopulmonary syndrome after liver transplantation. *Respiration* 1997; 6:173–175A.

11. Arguedas M, Abrams GA, Krowka MJ, Fallon MB. Prospective evaluation of outcomes and predictors of mortality in patients with hepatopulmonary syndrome undergoing liver transplantation. *Hepatology* 2003; 37:192–7.

12. Kaspar MD, Ramsay MA, Shuey CB, Levy MF, Klintmalm GG. Severe pulmonary hypertension and amelioration of hepatopulmonary syndrome after liver transplantation. *Liver Transpl Surg* 1998; 4:177–9.

13. Martinez-Palli G, Barbera JA, Taura P, Cirera I, Visa J, Rodriguez-Roisin R. Severe portopulmonary hypertension after liver transplantation in a patient with pre-existing hepatopulmonary syndrome. *J Hepatol* 1999; 31:1075–9.

14. Corley DA, Scharschmidt B, Bass N, Somberg K, Gold W. Lack of efficacy of TIPS for hepatopulmonary syndrome. *Gastroenterology* 1997; 113:728–31.

15. Mandell MS, Groves BM, Duke J. Progressive plexogenic pulmonary hypertension following liver transplantation. *Transplantation* 1995; 59:1488–90.

16. Abrams GA, Rose K, Fallon MB, McGuire BM, Bloomer JR, van Leeuwen DJ, et al. Hepatopulmonary syndrome and venous emboli causing intracerebral hemorrhages after liver transplantation: A case report. *Transplantation* 1999; 68:1–3.

17. Taille C, Cadranel J, Bellocq A, Thabut G, Soubrane O, Durand F, Ichai P, et al. Liver transplantation for hepatopulmonary syndrome: A ten-year experience in Paris, France. *Transplantation* 2003; 79:1482–9.

18. Collison EA, Nourmand H, Fraiman MH. Retrospective analysis of the results of liver transplantation for adults with severe hepatopulmonary syndrome. *Liver Transpl* 2002; 8:925–31.

19. Schiffer E, Majno P, Mentha G, Giostra E, Burri H, Klopfenstein E, et al. Hepatopulmonary syndrome increases the postoperative mortality rate following liver transplantation: A prospective study in 90 patients. *Am J Transpl* 2006; 6:1430–7.

20. http://www.unos.org.

21. Sulieman B, Voigt M, Katz D, Hunsicker L. Data driven policy for points allocation in hepatopulmonary syndrome. *Hepatology* 2005; 42:347A.

22. Schenk P, Fuhrmann V, Madl C, Funk G, Lehr S, Kandel O, Muller C. Hepatopulmonary syndrome: Prevalence and predictive value of various cut offs for arterial oxygenation and their clinical consequences. *Gut*. 2002; 51:853–9.

23. Krowka MJ, Mandell S, Ramsay MA, Kawut S, Fallon MB, Manzarbeitia C, Pardo M, et al. Hepatopulmonary syndrome and portopulmonary hypertension: A report of the Multicenter Liver Transplant Database. *Liver Transpl* 2004; 10:174–82.

24. Martinez G, Barbera J, Visa J, Rimola A, Parc J, Roca J, Navasa M, et al. Hepatopulmonary syndrome in candidates for liver transplantation. *J Hepatol* 2001; 34:756–8.

25. Abrams GA, Sanders MK, Fallon MB. Utility of pulse oximetry in the detection of arterial hypoxemia in liver transplant candidates. *Liver Transpl* 2002; 8:391–6.

26. Abrams GA, Jaffe CC, Hoffer PB, Binder HJ, Fallon MB. Diagnostic utility of contrast echocardiography and lung perfusion scan in patients with hepatopulmonary syndrome. *Gastroenterology* 1995; 109:1283–8.

27. Abrams G, Nanda N, Dubovsky E, Krowka M, Fallon M. Use of macroaggregated albumin lung perfusion scan to diagnose hepatopulmonary syndrome: A new approach. *Gastroenterology* 1998; 114: 305–10.

28. Abrams GA, Fallon MB. Treatment of hepatopulmonary syndrome with Allium sativum (garlic): A pilot trial. *J Clin Gastroenterol* 1998; 27:232–5.

29. Anel RM, Sheagren JN. Novel presentation and approach to management of hepatopulmonary syndrome with use of antimicrobial agents. *Clin Infect Dis* 2001; 32:E131–E136A.

30. Rabiller A, Nunes H, Lebrec D, Tazi KA, Wartski M, Dulmet E, et al. Prevention of Gram-negative translocation reduces the severity of hepatopulmonary syndrome. *Am J Respir Crit Care Med* 2002; 166:514–7.

31. Meyers C, Low L, Kaufman L, Druger G, Wong LL. Trendelenburg positioning and continuous lateral rotation improve oxygenation in hepatopulmonary syndrome after liver transplantation. *Liver Transpl Surg* 1998; 6:510–2.

32. Alexander J, Greenough A, Baker A, Rela M, Heaton N, Potter D. Nitric oxide treatment of severe hypoxemia after liver transplantation in hepatopulmonary syndrome. *Liver Transpl Surg* 1997; 3:54–5.

33. Durand P, Baujard C, Grosse AL. Reversal of hypoxemia by inhaled nitric oxide in children with severe hepatopulmonary syndrome, type 1, during and after liver transplantation. *Transplantation* 1998; 65:437–9.

8 Long-Term Metabolic Complications Posttransplantation
Controversies in Management

Lisa M. Forman, MD

CONTENTS

Abstract

Approximately 4,500 transplants are performed each year in the United States. Advances in organ preservation and surgical technique and in the management of immunosuppression have significantly improved survival. Short-term survival is excellent. As long-term survival increases, cardiovascular complications are emerging as a major cause of morbidity and mortality. Hypertension, dyslipidemia, and diabetes mellitus all are increased in liver transplant recipients and

From: *Clinical Gastroenterology: Liver Transplantation: Challenging Controversies and Topics*
Edited by: G. T. Everson and J. F. Trotter, DOI: 10.1007/978-1-60327-028-1_8,
© Humana Press, Totowa, NJ

occur at an earlier age than in the general population. As a result, they not only contribute to cardiovascular disease but also impact liver recipients' quality of life. Although primary care physicians claim to be comfortable in managing the care of liver recipients, transplant hepatologists usually assume these patients' overall health care. Many questions, however, need to be addressed regarding whom, in fact, is managing these metabolic complications and the adequacy of management. Ultimately, a novel health delivery system for liver recipients will need to be developed with the goal of improvement of quality of care.

Key Words: Liver transplantation; Metabolic complications; Hypertension; Dyslipidemia; Diabetes mellitus; Obesity; Osteoporosis

Liver transplantation has become the treatment of choice for many patients with end-stage liver disease. Approximately 4,500 transplants are performed each year in the United States. Advances in organ preservation and surgical technique and in the management of immunosuppression have significantly improved survival. Short-term survival is excellent, with overall one- and five-year patient survival rates of 87.5% and 73.9%, respectively (1). As long-term survival increases, cardiovascular complications are emerging as a major cause of morbidity and mortality. Recent data indicate that accelerated cardiovascular disease is second only to malignancy as a cause of late mortality (2).

As more liver transplant recipients survive into their first and second decades posttransplant, it is likely that more will develop metabolic complications and the metabolic syndrome. While prednisone is associated with diabetes and hypertension, and its withdrawal beneficial (3–5), little else is known about the genesis of the metabolic syndrome in this population. There are no guidelines for the treatment of cardiovascular complications in liver recipients, and it is unknown whether liver recipients are receiving adequate management. Looking for other risk factors for the development of metabolic complications is therefore crucial so that the transplant community can develop new strategies to aggressively modify cardiovascular risk factors to improve long-term survival.

BACKGROUND

It has been well recognized that accelerated cardiovascular disease is a leading cause of death and allograft loss in long-term survivors of both heart and kidney transplant recipients. The negative impact of cardiovascular disease on liver transplant recipients hasonly recently been addressed (6). In contrast to kidney and heart transplant candidates, liver transplant candidates have a low prevalence of cardiovascular risk factors prior to transplant. For this reason, liver recipients have traditionally been considered at low risk for cardiovascular complications posttransplant.

Many factors may predispose liver recipients to cardiovascular disease, including (1) use of immunosuppression, (2) change in lipoprotein metabolism induced by the new liver, and (3) changes in patient habits (diet, weight gain). For example, most immunosuppressive medications potentiate hypertension, dyslipidemia, and diabetes, but the root causes of metabolic complications largely remain unidentified (7, 8). Because of the magnitude of this problem, in 2001 an ad hoc group of transplant care physicians recommended that further research (including optimal management of dyslipidemia, defining cardiovascular disease progression rate) is needed (2).

Chronic renal insufficiency after liver transplantation is common and well recognized. Ojo et al., in a retrospective study using the Scientific Registry for Transplant Recipients, demonstrated that the one- and five-year risk of advanced chronic renal disease was 8% and 18.1%, respectively (9); renal failure often leads to increased morbidity and mortality (10, 11). The well-known association between calcineurin-inhibitor therapy and posttransplantation renal dysfunction (12) has led to the development of calcineurin-free immunosuppressive regimens. Despite the fact that even mild chronic renal insufficiency is associated with coronary artery disease, left ventricular hypertrophy, and congestive heart failure (13–15), the transplant community has not been as aggressive in managing other cardiovascular risk factors.

HYPERTENSION

Elevated blood pressure increases the risk for cardiovascular disease. Guidelines have been established for the general population, including more stringent diagnosis and treatment criteria in the setting of coexistent diabetes mellitus or chronic renal insufficiency (16).

The reported incidence of hypertension in liver transplant recipients has ranged from 40 to 85% (4, 17). However, the criteria for diagnosis of hypertension were not uniform across these reports, and in some cases only the prevalence of treated hypertension was reported. Hypertension is related to the use of glucocorticosteroids and calcineurin-inhibitors, perhaps by causing hypervolemia and renal afferent arteriole vasoconstriction, respectively (18).

DYSLIPIDEMIA

Dyslipidemia also increases cardiovascular disease risk, and guidelines have been established for the general population (19). Recent guidelines for renal transplant recipients advise a much more aggressive approach to its recognition and management (18). Dyslipidemia following liver transplantation has been reported to occur in 20–66% (4, 20, 21) and manifests primarily as hypertriglyceridemia as a side effect of immunosuppressive regimes, in particular sirolimus (8).

DIABETES MELLITUS

Diabetes and, to a similar extent, glucose intolerance and insulin resistance amplify other cardiovascular risk factors in the general population (22). New-onset diabetes mellitus results in increased susceptibility to infectious and cardiovascular complications and has a major impact on quality of life. Diabetes is associated with a two- to fourfold excess risk of cardiovascular disease (23, 24). Postliver transplantation diabetes is common, occurring in 5–35% (4, 17) of patients, with the majority of patients requiring insulin. Prior studies, however, have been difficult to interpret because of a lack of standardized definition of diabetes (23). Liver recipients are predisposed to develop diabetes because of immunosuppression, in particular glucocorticosteroids, and tacrolimus (25), as well as perhaps infection with hepatitis C (26). In addition, obesity, age, and ethnicity all contribute to increased risk for new-onset diabetes after transplantation (27). Hypertension and dyslipidemia also contribute to this increased risk. In the renal transplant population, posttransplant diabetes has clearly been associated with worse patient and allograft survival (25), but its impact on liver transplantation is less certain (28).

METABOLIC SYNDROME

The metabolic syndrome is a constellation of hypertension, glucose intolerance, dyslipidemia, and obesity (19, 29), with an overall prevalence of 22% in the general population (30). The prevalence increases with age and is highest among Hispanics (30). The mechanism underlying the metabolic syndrome is not fully known but is related to insulin resistance and leads to an increased risk of coronary disease and cardiovascular complications (31, 32).

Obesity is also quite common after liver transplantation, with reported rates of 20–50% (4, 17, 33). With the high prevalence of hypertension, dyslipidemia, and diabetes in this population as demonstrated above, liver recipients are predisposed to the metabolic syndrome. Because these risk factors are interlinked, tight control of all risk factors may be necessary to reduce posttransplant cardiovascular disease.

To date, no studies have directly addressed the issue of the metabolic syndrome in liver transplantation. Furthermore, prior studies regarding cardiovascular risk factors have been limited by small sample sizes, varying definitions of hypertension, dyslipidemia, and diabetes and often only report the prevalence of treated (versus uncontrolled or unrecognized) risk factors. Furthermore, which risk factors, and which risk score measurement in particular (i.e., Framingham risk score, etc.), are best in predicting future cardiovascular events is largely unknown (34).

OSTEOPOROSIS

Osteoporosis is also quite prevalent in liver recipients, with accelerated bone loss occurring in the first three to six months' posttransplantation. As a result, liver recipients are prone to fractures (occurring in 10–35%), predominantly of the ribs and vertebrae (35–37). Its pathogenesis is believed to be multifactorial and includes preexisting bone disease, prior history of alcoholism or cholestatic liver disease, vitamin D deficiency, secondary hyperparathyroidism, hypogonadism, immobility, and use of immunosuppressive agents, in particular glucocorticosteroids and calcineurin-inhibitors (38–40). With the use of newer immunosuppressive agents, and the avoidance of glucocorticosteroids, the current prevalence of osteoporosis, osteopenia, and fractures may be much lower. Diagnosing osteoporosis and therefore intervening before fractures occur may be challenging, as routine bone density measurements have not been shown to predict fracture risk and many insurance plans will not provide coverage for the testing (41). Despite the associated morbidity, a recent study, however, demonstrated that intravenous bisphosphonate treatment many prevent bone loss within the first year after liver transplantation (42).

METABOLIC COMPLICATION MANAGEMENT

With improved transplant outcomes, the cumulative volume of patients has grown (approximately 40,000 liver recipients are currently living in the United States) and what group of providers can best deliver optimal primary care has been debated. Although primary care physicians claim to be comfortable in managing the care of liver recipients, transplant hepatologists usually assume these patients' overall health care (43). Hepatologists, however, are not as comfortable as internists in managing cardiovascular complications, and probably don't do as good a job as primary care physicians in managing these complications. Anecdotally, liver recipients have expressed dissatisfaction with the care they are receiving from primary care physicians, whom they feel are hesitant to treat them and are unfamiliar with the immunosuppressive medications and potential drug–drug interactions. Primary care physicians have also acknowledged a knowledge deficit in the management of liver recipients. Furthermore, in the setting of chronic medical diseases (in this case "liver transplantation"), Redelmeier demonstrated that ancillary disorders are often undertreated (44).

To further investigate the issues regarding whom, in fact, is managing these metabolic complications and the perceived adequacy of their management, we conducted a study to determine attitudes, perceptions, and practice patterns in the management of metabolic complications after liver transplantation among hepatologists (45). Postal surveys were sent to all transplant hepatologists in the United States in programs that performed more than eight adult liver transplants in 2004. The response rate was 191 (68.2%) of 280 after accounting for incorrect addresses and physicians no longer in practice. The hepatologists' median age was 45 years (33–70); 85.5% were male, with median years since graduating from GI fellowship of 11 years (<1–39). Median center size was 64 (9–245) transplants per year. Liver recipients were assigned to a particular hepatologist in 42.7% of centers. Hepatologists, primary care physicians, and transplant surgeons were responsible for the overall care of recipients in 66%, 24.1%, and 8.4% of centers, respectively. The type of physician primarily responsible for the overall care of liver recipients was not associated with the center size or region. The majority of hepatologists indicated that they were comfortable in managing hypertension, chronic renal insufficiency, diabetes mellitus, dyslipidemia, and osteoporosis (84.8%, 71.5%, 61.9%, 76.2%, and 77.3%, respectively). Gender, center size, and years from fellowship were not associated with hepatologists' comfort level. Age was associated with comfort level in treating HTN (OR 0.94, $p = 0.011$). Most hepatologists felt that, ideally, primary care physicians should be managing recipients' hypertension, diabetes mellitus, dyslipidemia, and osteoporosis (78.9%, 63.3%, 78.3%, 72.5%), but felt that in actuality, primary care physicians are managing these conditions less frequently (45%, 51.4%, 44.6%, 38%).

Therefore, although there was some disagreement in what group of providers should be managing metabolic complications after liver transplantation, most hepatologists feel primary care physicians should take a more active role in the care of liver recipients.

It is imperative to further characterize the magnitude of cardiovascular risk factors in liver transplant recipients so that future prospective studies (both exploratory and interventional) can be performed with the goal of improvement of quality of care. Identifying barriers to care in the treatment of metabolic complications is crucial so that the transplant community can intervene to improve not only patient satisfaction and comfort level among primary care physicians, but also long-term survival. Further studies are needed to determine whether or not the liver transplant community is, in fact, doing an adequate job in managing metabolic complications and to determine barriers to primary care among liver recipients. A novel health delivery system for liver recipients will likely need to be developed with the goal of improvement of long-term survival.

CONCLUSION

As more and more people are living longer after liver transplantation, the prevalence of hypertension, diabetes mellitus, obesity, osteoporosis, and dyslipidemia will only increase. It is therefore crucial to have a better understanding of the prevalence of the posttransplant metabolic complications and the risk factors associated with them. Improving our understanding of these metabolic complications and our approach to their management has potential economic as well as scientific and clinical ramifications. The transplant community may need to change its focus from primarily treating rejection and avoiding calcineurin-inhibitors to aggressively managing hypertension, dyslipidemia, insulin resistance, diabetes, and obesity so as to improve not only renal function, but also overall survival.

REFERENCES

1. Annual report of the U.S. Scientific Registry for Transplant Recipients and the Organ and Procurement and Transplantation Network Transplant Data: 1989–1998. U.S. Department of Health and Human Services, Health Resources and Services Administration, Office of Special Programs, Division of Transplantation, Rockville, MD. UNOS, Richmond, VA.
2. Bostom AD, Brown RS, Cosio FG, et al. Prevention of post-transplant cardiovascular disease: Report and recommendations of an ad hoc group. *Am J Transpl* 2002; 2:491–500.
3. Everson GT, Trouillot T, Wachs M, et al. Early steroid withdrawal in liver transplantation is safe and beneficial. *Liver Transpl Surg* 1999; 5(Suppl 1):S48–S57.
4. Stegall MD, Everson G, Schroter G, Bilir B, Karrer F, Kam I. Metabolic complications after liver transplantation. *Transplantation* 1995; 60:1057–60.

5. Stegall MD, Everson GT, Schroter G, et al. Prednisone withdrawal late after adult liver transplantation reduces diabetes, hypertension, and hypercholesterolemia without causing graft loss. *Transpl Surg* 1997; 25:173–7.
6. Zeier M, Mandelbaum A, Ritz E. Hypertension in the transplanted patient. *Nephron* 1998; 80:257–68.
7. Lucey MR, Abdelmalek MF, Gagliardi R, et al. A comparison of tacrolimus and cyclosporine in liver transplantation: Effects on renal function and cardiovascular risk status. *Am J Transpl* 2005; 5:1111–9.
8. Trotter JF, Wachs ME, Trouillot TE, et al. Dyslipidemia during sirolimus therapy in liver transplant recipients occurs with concomitant cyclosporine but not tacrolimus. *Liver Transpl* 2001; 7:401–8.
9. Ojo AO, Held PJ, Port FK, et al. Chronic renal failure after transplantation of a nonrenal organ. *N Engl J Med* 2003; 348:931–40.
10. Brown RS, Lombardero M, Lake JR. Outcome of patients with renal insufficiency undergoing liver or liver-kidney transplantation. *Transplantation* 1996; 62:1788–93.
11. Rimola A, Gavaler JS, Schade RR, el-Lankany S, Starzl TE, Van Thiel DH. Effects of renal impairment on liver transplantation. *Gastroenterology* 1987; 93:148–56.
12. Porayko MK, Gonwa TA, Klintmalm GB, Wiesner RH. Comparing nephrotoxicity of FK 506 and cyclosporine regimens after liver transplantation: Preliminary results from U.S. Multicenter Trial. *Transpl Proc* 1995; 27:1114–6.
13. Fried LF, Shlipak MG, Crump C, et al. Renal insufficiency as a predictor of cardiovascular outcomes and mortality in elderly individuals. *J Am Coll Cardiol* 2003; 4:1364–72.
14. Shlipak MG, Heindenreich PA, Noguchi H, Chertow GM, Browner WS, McClellan, MB. Association of renal insufficiency with treatment and outcomes after myocardial infarction in elderly patients. *Ann Intern Med* 2002; 137:555–62.
15. Sarnak MJ, Levey AS. Cardiovascular disease and chronic renal disease: A new paradigm. *Am J Kidney Dis* 2000; 35(Suppl 1):S117–S131.
16. Chobanian AV, Bakris GL, Black HR, et al. Seventh report of the Joint National Committee on prevention, detection, evaluation, and treatment of high blood pressure. *Hypertension* 2003; 42:1206–52.
17. Sheiner PA, Magliocca JF, Bodian CA, et al. Long-term medical complications in patients surviving $\geq$ 5 years after liver transplant. *Transplantation* 2000; 69:781–9.
18. National Kidney Foundation Work Group. Clinical practice guidelines for managing dyslipidemias in kidney transplant patients: A report from the Managing Dyslipidemias in Chronic Kidney Disease Work Group of the National Kidney Foundation Kidney Disease Outcomes Quality Initiative. *Am J Transpl* 2004; 4:13–53.
19. Expert Panel on Detection, Evaluation, and Treatment of High Blood Cholesterol in Adults. Executive Summary of the Third Report of the National Cholesterol Education Program (NCEP) Expert Panel on Detection, Evaluation, and Treatment of High Blood Cholesterol in Adults (Adult Treatment Panel III). *JAMA* 2001; 285:2486–97.

20. Munoz SJ, Doems RO, Moritz MJ, Martin P, Jarrell BE, Maddrey WC. Hyper-lipidemia and obesity after orthotopic liver transplantation. *Transpl Proc* 1991; 23:1480–3.

21. Gisbert C, Prieto M, Berenguer M, et al. Hyperlipidemia in liver transplant recipients: Prevalence and risk factors. *Liver Transpl Surg* 1997; 3:416–23.

22. Stamler J, Vaccaro O, Neaton JD, Wentworth D. Diabetes, other risk factors, and 12 years cardiovascular mortality for men screened in the Multiple Risk Factor Intervention Trial. *Diabetes Care* 1993; 16:434–44.

23. The Expert Committee on the Diagnosis and Classification of Diabetes Mellitus: Report of the Expert Committee on the Diagnosis and Classification of Diabetes Mellitus. *Diabetes Care* 1997; 20:1183–97.

24. The Expert Committee on the Diagnosis and Classification of Diabetes Mellitus: Follow-up report on the diagnosis of diabetes mellitus. *Diabetes Care* 2003; 26:3160–7.

25. Kasiske BL, Snyder JJ, Gilbertson D, Matas AJ. Diabetes mellitus after kidney transplantation in the United States. *Am J Transpl* 2003; 3:178–85.

26. Khalili M, Lim JW, Bass N, Ascher NL, Roberts JP, Terrault NA. New onset diabetes mellitus after liver transplantation: The critical role of hepatitis C infection. *Liver Transpl* 2004; 10:349–55.

27. Davidson JA, Wilkinson A. New-Onset Diabetes After Transplantation 2003 International Consensus Guidelines: An endocrinologist's view. *Diabetes Care* 2004; 27:805–12.

28. Trail KC, McCashland TM, Larse JL, et al. Morbidity in patients with posttransplant diabetes mellitus following orthotopic liver transplantation. *Liver Transpl Surg* 1996; 2:276–83.

29. Alberti KG, Zimmet PZ. Definition, diagnosis and classification of diabetes mellitus and its complications. Part 1: Diagnosis and classification of diabetes mellitus provisional report of a WHO consultation. *Diabetes Med* 1998; 15:539–53.

30. Ford ES, Giles WH, Dietz WH. Prevalence of the metabolic syndrome among US adults: Findings from the Third National Health and Nutrition Examination Survey. *JAMA* 2002; 287:356–9.

31. DeFronzo RA, Ferrannini E. Insulin resistance: A multifaceted syndrome responsible for NIDDM, obesity, hypertension, dyslipidemia, and atherosclerotic cardiovascular disease. *Diabetes Care* 1991; 14:173–94.

32. Lakka HM, Laaksonen DE, Lakka TA, et al. The metabolic syndrome and total and cardiovascular disease mortality in middle-aged men. *JAMA* 2002; 288:2709–16.

33. Everhart JE, Lombardero M, Lake JR, Wiesner RH, Zetterman RK, Hoofnager JH. Weight change and obesity after liver transplantation: Incidence and risk factors. *Liver Transpl Surg* 1998; 4:285–96.

34. Guckelberger O, Mutzke F, Glanemann M, et al. Validation of cardiovascular risk scores in a liver transplant population. *Liver Transpl* 2006; 12:394–401.

35. Diamond T, Stiel D, Wilkinson M, Riche J, Posen S. Osteoporosis and skeletal fractures in chronic liver disease. *Gut* 1990; 31:82–7.

36. Monegal A, Navasa M, Guanabens N, et al. Bone disease after liver transplantation: A long-term prospective study of bone mass changes, hormonal status and histomorphometric characteristics. *Osteoporosis Int* 2001; 12:484–92.

37. Compston JE. Osteoporosis after liver transplantation. *Liver Transpl* 2003; 9:321–30.
38. Hay JE. Osteoporosis in liver diseases and after liver transplantation. *J Hepatol* 2003; 38:856–86.
39. Segal E, Baruch Y, Kramsky R, Raz B, Tamir A, Ish-Shalom S. Predominant factors associated with bone loss in liver transplant patients after prolonged post-transplantation period. *Clin Transpl* 2003; 17:13–9.
40. Smallwood GA, Burns D, Fasola CG, Steiber AC, Heffron TG. Relationship between immunosuppression and osteoporosis in an outpatient liver transplant clinic. *Transpl Proc* 2005; 37:1910–1.
41. Hardinger KL, Ho B, Schnitzler MA, et al. Serial measurements of bone density at the lumbar spine do not predict fracture risk after liver transplantation. *Liver Transpl* 2003; 9:857–62.
42. Crawford BAL, Kam C, Pavlovic J, et al. Zoledronic acid prevents bone loss after liver transplantation. *Ann Intern Med* 2006; 144:239–48.
43. McCashland TM. Posttransplantation care: Role of primary care physician versus transplant center. *Liver Transpl* 2001; 7:S2–S12.
44. Redelmeier DA, Tan SH, Booth GL. The treatment of unrelated disorders in patients with chronic medical diseases. *N Engl J Med* 1998; 338:1516–20.
45. Forman LM, Osborne JC, Everson GT. Long-term management after liver transplantation: Primary care physician vs. hepatologist? *Am J Transpl* 2006; p. 2031A.

9 Hepatitis B and Liver Transplantation
Current Trends

Geoffrey McCaughan, MBBS, MD, FRACP, PhD, Jade D. Jamias, MD, FPCP, DPSG, DPSDE, Qingchun Fu, MD, Nicholas Shackel, MBBS, MD, FRACP, PhD, and Simone Strasser, MBBS, MD, FRACP

CONTENTS

Abstract

Over 300 million people are infected with the hepatitis B virus (HBV); of these, approximately 20% will develop cirrhosis and

From: *Clinical Gastroenterology: Liver Transplantation: Challenging Controversies and Topics*
Edited by: G. T. Everson and J. F. Trotter, DOI: 10.1007/978-1-60327-028-1_9,
© Humana Press, Totowa, NJ

complications of end-stage liver disease including hepatocellular carcinoma. Thus, liver transplantation has emerged as an important therapy for selected patients with HBV infection. The authors review the management of HBV before and after liver transplantation, which has become more complex with the advent of several new efficacious oral therapies over the past few years. In addition, the outcomes for HBV patients after liver transplantation are reviewed along with the use of hepatitis B immune globulin (HBIg). Finally, the authors speculate on the possibility of oral therapies supplanting long-term HBIg administration.

Key Words: Hepatitis B; Hepatocellular carcinoma; Hepatitis B immunoglobulin; Lamivudine; Adefovir; Hepatitis B vaccination

BURDEN OF DISEASE

Worldwide, an estimated 350 million people are chronically infected with the hepatitis B virus (HBV) (1). Without antiviral treatment, approximately 20% will develop cirrhosis and complications of end-stage liver disease (2, 3). HBV-related liver failure accounts for about one million deaths per year (4, 5). Furthermore, chronic HBV infection is a major risk factor for hepatocellular carcinoma (HCC). The relative risk of HCC among HBV carriers is 100-fold times greater than in hepatitis B surface antigen (HBsAg)-negative persons (6). Thus, liver transplantation has emerged as an important therapy for select patients with HBV infection.

INDICATIONS FOR LIVER TRANSPLANTATION

The indications for liver transplantation for hepatitis B are the same as those for other causes of liver disease, such as fulminant hepatic failure (FHF), hepatic decompensation in a patient with established cirrhosis, or HCC.

In 1997, the United Network for Organ Sharing (UNOS) established a CP score of 7 or higher as the minimal listing criteria for eligibility of listing for liver transplantation (LT) (Table 1) (7). A CTP score of 7 or higher equates to an estimated 90% or lower chance of one-year survival without transplantation. However, single clinical features such as ascites or encephalopathy may occasionally direct decision making. In the United States, the Model for End-Stage Liver Disease (MELD) scoring system has become an evidence-based means of organ allocation (8). The MELD score is a severity score predictive of mortality in

Table 1
Scoring System for Determining Severity for Hepatitis B-Associated Cirrhosis

Child–Pugh Score	1	2	3
Encephalopathy	None	Grade 1–2	Grade 3–4
Ascites	Absent	Slight	Moderate/marked
Bilirubin (mg/dL)	<2	2–3	>3
Albumin (g/L)	>35	28–35	<28
INR	<1.7	1.7–2.3	>2.3
MELD Score	$\log_e$Bilirubin (mg/dL) + $\log_e$creatinine (mg/dL) + $\log_e$INR		

INR = international normalized ratio; MELD = Model for End-stage Liver Disease.

patients with chronic liver disease (9, 10). Recent data have indicated that the greatest proportion of patients receiving liver transplantation in 2001–2003 had a MELD score of 15 to 17. The same data suggested a survival benefit from transplantation only if the MELD score was 18 or higher (11). Because the MELD system was not affected by HCC, a prioritization system was developed that allows selected patients with HCC to undergo transplantation.

PRETRANSPLANT ANTIVIRAL THERAPY

Studies have shown that active HBV replication prior to orthotopic liver transplantation (OLT) is the main risk factor for disease recurrence. In the absence of preventive therapies, liver transplantation for patients with either acute or chronic replicating HBV infection resulted in universal reinfection of the allograft, progressive graft failure, and increased mortality even with retransplantation (12–14). Consequently, therapeutic strategies to reduce or eliminate HBV replication prior to OLT should lower the incidence of reinfection.

Characteristics of an ideal antiviral agent(s) include a wide margin of safety and low toxicity in the setting of decompensated cirrhosis and a rapid ability to eliminate HBV replication in patients with either acute or chronic infections. Until recently, the only treatment for chronic hepatitis B was standard interferon (IFN). Unfortunately, IFN has limited efficacy and may be associated with severe sepsis and worsening of hepatic failure in patients with decompensated cirrhosis (15, 16).

Over the last decade, the availability of several nucleoside/nucleotide analogues has significantly changed the management of end-stage liver disease caused by HBV. Nucleoside analogues inhibit HBV DNA polymerase by binding to its active site, but as with most antiviral drugs, they do not eradicate the covalently closed circular DNA (ccDNA) (17).

Lamivudine

Lamivudine (LAM) has been extensively studied in OLT candidates (Table 2). It is usually given at 100 mg daily, with dose adjustments in the presence of renal failure. It is safe and well tolerated in decompensated cirrhosis and results in undetectable HBV DNA using molecular hybridization in 63–100% of patients in two to three months. Available evidence showed that it improves the Child–Pugh Score (CPS) and decreases the need for hospital admission for resistant ascites, spontaneous bacterial peritonitis (SBP), and encephalopathy (18, 19). Moreover, clinical and biochemical improvements are not limited to HBe-positive patients but are noted in HBe-negative-associated cirrhosis as well.

The impact of LAM therapy for three to six months prior to OLT on hepatic function and transplant-free survival has been analyzed in several studies (19–25). Data from these studies showed that LAM can stabilize patients on the waiting list, allowing them to proceed to transplant as well as reducing the risk of disease recurrence posttransplant. However, HCC can still occur even among those with significant clinical improvement, and continued surveillance is thus required.

It has also been shown that continuous treatment with LAM delays clinical progression in patients with compensated HBV cirrhosis by significantly reducing the incidence of hepatic decompensation and the risk of HCC. The magnitude of protection is substantial, with a reduction of approximately 50% in disease progression during a median period of 32 months of treatment (26). Although many patients derived clinical benefits from LAM, there is a subgroup of patients who present with rapidly progressive disease in whom fatal outcomes are seen despite the introduction of LAM.

Fontana and associates (22) showed in a multivariate model that pretreatment serum bilirubin and creatinine levels as well as the presence of detectable HBV DNA by branched DNA assay were significantly associated with poor six-month survival. Altogether, these data indicate that there may be a subpopulation of individuals with extremely advanced disease who require urgent transplantation and do not benefit from LAM treatment.

Table 2
Results of Lamivudine Therapy for Hepatitis B Virus-Related Decompensated Cirrhosis

Authors	Year	Number of Patients	Follow-up Duration (months)	Number (%) of Patients with Improvement in CPS	Number (%) of Patients Trans-planted	Number (%) of Deaths
Villeneuve et al. (18)	2000	35	19	22 (63%)	8 (23%)	7 (20%)
Kapoor et al. (24)	2000	18	17.9	(50%)	0 (0%)	0 (0%)
Yao et al. (19)	2001	23	13	14 (60.9%)	(34.8%)	0 (0%)
Perrillo et al. (20)	2001	77	38	NA	47 (61%)	0 (0%)
Hann et al. (25)	2001	70	13.3	NA	NA	NA
Fontana et al. (21)	2002	162	6	NA	91 (56%)	18 (11%)

CPS = Child–Pugh Score; NA = not available.

Another major concern in addition to the issue of early LAM failure is the emergence of LAM resistance due to one or more mutations in the YMDD motif of the HBV DNA polymerase gene that can be detected in 15–30% of patients after one year and in up to 70% after five years of continued treatment (27, 28). HBV DNA and serum ALT levels often remain lower than baseline when resistance is first diagnosed. However, HBV DNA levels increase and hepatitis flares occur with increasing frequency over time due to the selection of compensatory mutations (29). Hepatitis flares associated with breakthrough infection may result in rapid hepatic decompensation, leading to death in the absence of semi-urgent transplantation. Patients with underlying cirrhosis are at particularly high risk for such complications (30). In this situation, treatment with adefovir (ADV) (10 mg daily) may be associated with rapid decrease in HBV DNA and progressive clinical improvement. Although adefovir therapy is safe and well tolerated, some patients fail to improve quickly enough to avoid liver transplantation.

Presently, an increasing number of patients with chronic hepatitis B-associated liver failure are undergoing transplantation with either genotypic or phenotypic LAM resistance. Thus, a significant number of patients are going to transplantation on combined LAM and ADV therapy or on ADV monotherapy.

POSTTRANSPLANT ANTIVIRAL THERAPY

Monotherapy: Hepatitis B Immune Globulin (HBIg)

In the late 1980s in Europe and the early 1990s in the United States, the use of passive immunoprophylaxis with HBIg resulted in a significant reduction in the incidence of recurrent HBV. The mechanism by which HBIg monotherapy controls recurrence of disease is poorly understood. It has been hypothesized that it protects naïve hepatocytes against HBV released from extrahepatic sites by blocking a putative HBV receptor (35); alternatively, it may neutralize circulating virions through immune precipitation and immune complex formation (36).

Results from studies involving patients with autoimmune disorders suggest that HBIg may have immune regulatory functions (31, 32). Patients on long-term HBIg immunoprophylaxis have a much lower incidence of rejection as compared with other indications for OLT, with the exception of alcoholic liver disease (33). Moreover, some form of HBIg-associated immune suppression or tolerance has been observed in some post-OLT patients. In these patients, HBV DNA is present in hepatocytes, but there is no evidence of host inflammatory response, hepatocellular injury, or circulating virus (34).

HBIg is administered first during the anhepatic phase of OLT; subsequent dose regimens are designed to maintain an effective titer of opsonizing anti-HBs. The most common regimen consists of 10,000 IU given intravenously during the anhepatic phase and then daily for the first eight post-op days and every one to three months thereafter. Immediately post-OLT, the level of circulating HBV is high; thus, a target trough level of 500 IU/L has been recommended (37). Later in the posttransplant course, replication from extrahepatic sites becomes the source of HBV, for which a lower trough level of 100–150 IU/L has been considered protective if maintained indefinitely (37, 38).

In the large European multicenter study by Samuel et al. (39), the rate of recurrent infection was directly related to the amount of replication before and after OLT, being least in those transplanted for fulminant hepatitis B (17%) and greatest in cirrhotics (67%). Reinfection among patients with replicative HBV infection (HBV DNA-positive or HBe-positive) pre-OLT occurred in 83% ± 6%; these patients were given higher doses of HBIg to maintain anti-HBs levels greater than 500 IU/L. The role of HBIg in preventing graft HBV reinfection has been observed repeatedly in subsequent studies (40–44).

HBIg is safe and well tolerated, but mild to moderate adverse events have been observed. Hypersensitivity reaction or even anaphylaxis may occur rarely as with other immune globulins (35).

HBIg therapy has two major drawbacks:

1. It is expensive, and IV preparation is unavailable in most transplant centers. This has led to the use of intramuscular HBIg. However, due to the small number of patients studied and the short duration of follow-up of the different studies, there is limited experience on the effectiveness of this route.
2. Therapy must be maintained on a long-term basis or possibly indefinitely. Discontinuation, even several years posttransplantation, resulted in most cases in the reappearance of HBV in the graft. Furthermore, the immune pressure exerted by anti-HBs may lead to the selection of surface antigen mutants, resulting in allograft reinfection.

Monotherapy: Lamivudine

Lamivudine prevents allograft reinfection by inhibiting replication of HBV in extrahepatic sites (Table 3). Several studies have investigated the efficacy of pre- and post-OLT LAM therapy to prevent recurrent HBV infection without the need for additional HBIg prophylaxis (20, 45–48). Results were encouraging, with reappearance of HBs Ag in the serum of 18–32% of patients after 6 to 16 months of follow-up. The

Table 3
Efficacy of Lamivudine Monotherapy Pre- and Post-Orthotic Liver Transplantation

Authors	Year	Number of Patients	Number of Patients HBV DNA-Positive Pre-OLT	Number of Patients HBeAg-Positive Pre-OLT	Mean Duration of LAM Therapy Pre-OLT (Months)	Number of Patients Transplanted	Number (%) of Patients with HBV Recurrence
Grellier et al. (45)	1996	17	8	4	2	12	5 (50%)
Mutimer et al. (46)	2000	23	9	11	NA	17	5 (29.4%)
Malkan et al. (47)	2000	13	3	2	8	13	4 (30.7%)
Perrillo et al. (20)	2001	77	26	24	2.1	47	17 (36.1%)
Lo et al. (48)	2001	31	11	18	1.6	31	7 (22.6%)

OLT = orthotopic liver transplantation; NA = not available.

overall reinfection rate ranged from 22.6% in Lo et al.'s group (48) to 50% in Grellier et al.'s group (45). Breakthrough infection with YMDD mutants accounted for the majority of HBV recurrence (23–50% of patients) and increased mortality in some patients. Moreover, a strong association between the status of viral replication before treatment and the risk of graft reinfection was demonstrated. Mutimer and associates further suggested that a high pre-LAM serum HBV titer may predict subsequent post-OLT emergence of YMDD variant HBV.[46]

Interestingly, 42% (21 of 50) of Lo et al.'s cohort who became HBsAg-negative with LAM monoprophylaxis spontaneously developed anti-HBs. The peak anti-HBs titer was found within three months after transplantation and exceeded 100 mIU/mL in more than 50% of the cases. They hypothesized that this antibody is probably produced by functional lymphocytes transferred from the donor to the recipient, suggesting the possibility of adoptive transfer of immunity from the liver graft. Although the results on this novel concept appear promising, further studies are needed to determine the durability of anti-HBs production as well as long-term protective efficacy, since the majority of the cohort had a declining anti-HBs titer over time.

At present, LAM monotherapy appears to be inadequate prophylaxis for recurrent HBV infection and, therefore, cannot be recommended except in the situation of passively transferred anti-HBs from the donor.

Combination Therapy: Hepatitis B Immune Globulin and Lamivudine

Clearly, HBIg or LAM monotherapy against HBV has improved survival and decreased the likelihood of disease recurrence in HBV-infected LT recipients. The emergence of LAM-resistant YMDD mutants after prolonged LAM monotherapy and the high recurrence rate with HBIg monotherapy among patients with replicative HBV infection pre-OLT have provided the rationale for using combination therapy as a means of preventing HBV recurrence among LT recipients (Table 4).

Possible mechanisms for the efficacy of combined HBIg and LAM include the synergy of (1) LAM decreasing the viral load, which may prevent saturation of HBIg binding sites and thus reduce the immune pressure, leading to the emergence of surface gene mutations, (2) HBIg preventing receptor-mediated entry of HBV into hepatocytes and extrahepatic cells required for the production of escape mutations in the YMDD motif (49, 54).

The combination of LAM therapy pre- and post- with HBIg post-OLT has become the standard of care in most liver transplant centers.

Table 4
Efficacy of Combination Therapy of Lamivudine and HBIg in the Prevention of HBV Recurrence After Liver Transplantation

Authors	Year	Number of Patients	Number of Patients HBV-DNA-Positive Pre-OLT	Number of Patients HBeAg-Positive Pre-OLT	Duration LAM Treatment Pre-OLT (Months)	HBIg Route	Number (%) of Patients with HBV Recurrence
Markowitz et al. (52)	1998	14	5	1	3	IV	0 (0%)
Yao et al. (55)	1999	10	9	6	8.6	IV then IM	1 (10%)
Yoshida et al. (56)	1999	7	4	NA	NA	IM	0 (0%)
McCaughan et al. (57)	1999	9	9	0	0	IM	0 (0%)
Angus et al. (51)	2000	37	36	19	3.2	IM	1 (3%)
Han et al. (49)	2000	59	NA	NA	NA	IV	0 (0%)
Marzano et al. (50)	2001	33	26	7	4.6	IV	1 (4%)
Seehofer et al. (53)	2001	17	17	9	10.6	IV	3 (18%)
Rosenau et al. (54)	2001	21	11	3	4.6	IV	2 (9.5%)
Gane et al. (93)	2002	107	79	39	2	IM	4 (4%)
Roche et al. (41)	2003	15	15	5	4.6	IV	1 (6.6%)
Lilly et al. (58)	2005	43	NA	NA	NA	IV	3 (7%)

HBIg = Hepatitis B immune globulin; HBeAg = Hepatitis Be antigen; OLT = orthotopic liver transplantation; LAM = lamivudine; IM = intramuscular; IV = intravenous; NA = not available.

Many series showed that the mean reinfection rate was only 5.2% (range 0–18%) after one to two years (41, 49–57). Han et al. (49) found that combination therapy was more cost-effective when compared to HBIg therapy alone. It resulted in an average cost savings of $24,786 per patient and an average cost-effectiveness ratio (ACER) of $252,111 per recurrence prevented compared to $362,570 per recurrence prevented with the monotherapy strategy.

The efficacy was similarly shown in several studies involving low-dose HBIg protocols (51, 54, 55, 58). Transplant centers such as the authors' in Australia and in New Zealand use a very low dose of HBIg (400–800 units intramuscularly) to maintain an anti-HBs titer between 50–100 IU/L. This protocol results in a very low recurrence rate under 5% (51).

At present, the use of LAM and low-dose HBIg therapy appears as a safe and effective strategy against HBV recurrence among LT recipients. However, the question of whether there is a need for a higher dose of HBIg for patients with high viral load or those with LAM-resistant mutants at the time of transplantation is still to be determined.

Combination Therapy: Lamivudine and Adefovir

The protective effect of LAM prophylaxis on post-OLT HBV recurrence is incomplete in viremic patients. This loss of efficacy is frequently related to selection of YMDD mutants (39, 59, 60). The emergence of these mutants pre-OLT has been associated with recurrence of hepatitis B disease despite combination therapy with HBIg and LAM (54).

The incidence of pretransplanation YMDD mutants is increasing and is expected to increase further in the near future. Thus, an effective alternative prophylactic strategy for these patients is of prime importance.

Adefovir dipivoxil is the prodrug of adefovir, a nucleotide analogue against HBV-DNA polymerase. It has both *in vitro* (61) and *in vivo* (62) efficacy against both wild-type and LAM-resistant HBV. In contrast to LAM, resistance to ADV appears to be delayed and infrequent (67, 68) and viral mutants resistant to ADV remain sensitive to LAM. This lack of cross-resistance (61) between LAM and ADV suggests that combination of these two drugs may be the superior approach in patients with LAM resistance to prevent the development of multidrug-resistant HBV viral strains.

Lok et al. recently showed that the cumulative probability of adefovir resistance mutations among OLT patients at one, two, and three years is 1.5%, 13.3%, and 13.3%, respectively, and that factors associated with resistance include the use of ADV monotherapy and HBV genotype D (63).

To date, the largest published study of the use of ADV for the treatment of LAM-resistant HBV in the pre- and posttransplant setting was by Schiff et al. (64). It involved 324 subjects, all of whom had detectable HBV DNA despite LAM therapy. Improvement in the virological, biochemical, and clinical profiles were observed in pre- and post-OLT patients with the addition of ADV. Likewise, there was stabilization or improvement in the CPS of both groups. After one year of therapy, survival was 84% in the pre-LT group and 93% in the post-LT group. The subsequent studies of Perillo et al. (65) and Lo et al. (66) on the efficacy of add-on ADV to LAM confirmed these findings.

One major issue with the use of ADV is nephrotoxicity. The incidence of ADV-associated nephrotoxicity during the course of HBV treatment appears to be lower. However, concomitant nephrotoxic medications (i.e., calcineurin-inhibitors) or prior renal injury may limit its use in the transplant population (67).

CAN HBIG BE DISCONTINUED?

As mentioned earlier, one of the major downsides of HBIg immunoprophylaxis is the need to administer it on a long-term or probably indefinite basis, which adds considerably to an already very expensive procedure, not to mention the inconvenience of administration.

The feasibility of HBIg discontinuation at various intervals following OLT has been examined in several studies, which we describe next.

LAM Monotherapy After HBIg Withdrawal or After Combined HBIg/LAM

Two studies examined the reinfection rate after HBIg withdrawal followed by LAM monotherapy. In the series by Dodson et al. (70), 16 HBeAg-negative patients at the time of OLT remained HBsAg-negative after a mean follow-up of 13 months. Naoumov and colleagues (71) randomized 24 pre-OLT HBV DNA-negative patients to receive LAM monotherapy or continue with passive immunoprophylaxis with HBIg. The graft reinfection rates at week 52 were 16.6% and 8.3%, respectively.

Discontinuation of HBIg following combination therapy HBIg and LAM has also been explored. Buti et al. (72) randomized 29 patients who were HBV DNA-negative at the time of OLT (12 spontaneously and 17 LAM-induced) to receive LAM monotherapy or combination therapy of HBIg and LAM one month post-OLT. None of the patients developed clinical reinfection during 18 months of observation. In the series of Terrault et al. (73), none of the patients who were converted to LAM monotherapy after 6 months of combined HBIg and LAM therapy developed recurrence after a median follow-up of 13.8 months post-OLT.

Results of these studies tend to suggest that the use of LAM after HBIg withdrawal and especially the use of combination prophylaxis followed by LAM monotherapy may be a more expedient and cost-effective strategy to prevent recurrent HBV after OLT. However, despite the apparent advantage of convenience and cost reduction, it should be noted that all the studies that examined the efficacy of this strategy involved low-risk patients (i.e., HBeAg-negative, HBV DNA-negative). Furthermore, HBIg withdrawal still poses a risk since there are no definite tests to identify patients who have cleared HBV from liver and plasma, and, once reinfection occurs, HBIg therapy is not effective.

Further studies are needed to determine the optimal timing of HBIg withdrawal and to investigate whether this alternative approach is applicable to high-risk patients.

Vaccination After or During HBIg Withdrawal

HBV vaccination is highly effective in healthy individuals, with a seroconversion rate higher than 90% (74–76). However, results among immunosuppressed patients have been disappointing (77). The seroconversion rate is very low among patients who were transplanted for non-HBV-related cirrhosis and chronic hepatitis C (78–80). Previous anecdotal reports on the failure of vaccination among patients transplanted for hepatitis B liver failure are also available.

The use of active immunization to obviate the need for long-term HBIg has been investigated in several studies. Sanchez-Fueyo et al. (81, 82) and Bienzle et al. (83) showed that in a selected group of liver transplant recipients, HBIg immunoprophylaxis can safely be discontinued after inducing anti-HBs seroconversion with HBV vaccination. Seroconversion was noted in 80% and 50% of patients, respectively. However, the anti-HBs titer achieved was low in most patients and may not be protective.

These promising results were not confirmed in the series of Angelico et al. (84) wherein anti-HBs seroconversion was observed in only 17.6% of patients despite administration of the vaccine not only through the conventional intramuscular route, but also intradermally.

To enhance the immune response to vaccination, studies using novel adjuvant systems were explored. One such study by Starkel et al. (85) evaluated the immunogenicity of a novel adjuvant, 3-deacylated

monophosphoryl lipid A (MPL) in 15 liver transplant patients: 10 transplanted for HBV and 5 transplanted for non-viral-related liver diseases.
Response rates were 40% (4 of 10) and 80% (4 of 5), respectively. Although the titer of antiHBs reached for HBV group was much lower
(>500 IU/L vs. >1,000 IU/L), discontinuation of HBIg prophylaxis for
almost three years after vaccination was allowed in all of the responders.

HBV vaccination using standard preparation or vaccines formulated
with immunostimulatory adjuvants appears to be safe and may allow
long-term discontinuation of HBIg in selected patients, thereby saving
a considerable amount of financial resources. However, the available
data for this attractive strategy are preliminary and conflicting. There is
still a great need for future studies to look into the optimal vaccination
schedule, to determine ways to improve the vaccination regimen, and to
identify factors associated with increased response rate to vaccination.

Posttransplant De Novo HBV Infection

The increasing disparity between liver allograft supply and demand
has led to the use of livers from donors with evidence of past hepatitis
B infection, i.e., those who are HBV core antibody-positive and HBs
antigen-negative.

LT recipients of anti-HBc-positive donors are at risk for de novo
HBV infection because immunosuppression may lead to HBV reactivation (86, 87). The risk of HBV transmission is highest for anti-HBc-
negative and anti-Hbs-negative recipients in the absence of prophylaxis
(88). HBIg monotherapy (89), LAM monotherapy (90, 99), and combination therapy of HBIg and LAM (91) have all been used effectively in
this setting.

Presently, many transplant centers preferentially offer the use of such
donor livers to HBsAg-positive or anti-HBs-positive recipients. However, de novo infection may still be observed in the latter group, indicating that antiviral prophylaxis may still be required.

OUTCOMES OF LIVER TRANSPLANTATION
FOR HBV-RELATED LIVER DISEASE

With the development of several effective antiviral prophylaxes
against HBV recurrence in the transplant setting, the outcomes of liver
transplantation for HBV-related liver failure are now excellent and allograft infection poses a relatively minor threat to long-term survival.

In a recent report by Kim et al. (92), in the United States, the one- and
five-year survival rates for patients transplanted for HBV-related liver

failure were 87% and 76%, respectively. Patient outcomes, adjusting for other variables, were comparable with, if not slightly better than, those patients with other etiologies of liver failure. Furthermore, the improvement in patient survival underscores the effectiveness of the different therapeutic strategies that have been adopted in the past two decades and indicates timely and widespread use of these measures by transplant centers in the United States.

FUTURE DIRECTIONS

Several studies have shown that patients with nonreplicative HBV infection at the time of OLT are at the lowest risk of HBV recurrence after transplant. Therefore, the development of new oral antiviral agents will definitely broaden the therapeutic armamentarium for eliminating HBV replication prior to OLT either used alone or in combination. Preliminary studies on new nucleoside analogues, i.e., entecavir (94, 95) and tenofovir (96–98), are now being undertaken, but their role in the treatment of HBV in the transplant setting is still to be determined. If effective oral drugs are developed, the use of passive immunoprophylaxis with HBIg will likely be limited to patients with residual HBV DNA at the time of OLT (Table 5).

Further development of HBV vaccines, especially those that incorporate pre-S antigens and immunostimulatory adjuvants that are more immunogenic, may permit effective immunization of liver transplant recipients. Furthermore, the transplant community might be able to consider a broader use of organs from hepatitis B core antigen antibody-positive donors for patients who respond to vaccination and can potentially provide an additional means of extending the donor pool, especially so in this era of organ shortage.

Table 5
Likely Future Approaches

Pretransplant	Commence combination therapies
	– ? Lamivudine/adefovir
	– ? Entacavir/tenofovir
	– ? Lamivudine/tenofovir
Posttransplant	Continue combination therapy with early HBIg withdrawal

HBIg = Hepatitis B immune globulin; HBeAg = Hepatitis Be antigen; OLT = orthotopic liver transplantation; LAM = lamivudine; IM = intramuscular; IV = intravenous; NA = not available.

CONCLUSIONS

Hepatitis B virus-related liver failure with or without hepatocellular carcinoma is one of the major indications for liver transplantation. Among patients with decompensated hepatitis B cirrhosis, LAM therapy is highly effective in suppressing HBV replication and has significantly improved clinical outcomes. However, prolonged therapy has been frequently complicated by the emergence of YMDD mutants, which cause breakthrough infection, leading to rapid hepatic decompensation requiring urgent transplantation or death. Adefovir dipivoxil is a safe and effective agent against LAM-resistant mutants.

Antiviral agents should be given to patients with HBV-related liver disease pre- and post-OLT to prevent allograft infection, particularly to those considered high-risk. To date, LAM monotherapy cannot be recommended as adequate prophylaxis for HBV recurrence. Combination therapy with HBIg and LAM appears to be the most effective strategy of preventing recurrent HBV infection following liver transplantation. HBIg withdrawal followed by LAM monotherapy or active immunization is an attractive alternative for prophylaxis against recurrent HBV disease in those with very low HBV DNA at the commencement of therapy (Fig. 1).

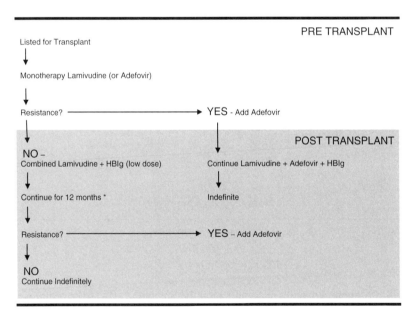

Fig. 1. Current recommendations. For low-risk group (HBV DNA-negative, HBeAg-negative), recent studies have shown that it may be possible to withdraw HBIg and maintain patients on lamivudine or give active immunization, but this still requires further study.

REFERENCES

1. World Health Organization. Hepatitis B fact sheet. October 2000.
2. Fattovich G. Natural history of hepatitis B. *J Hepatol* 2003; 39:50–8.
3. Liaw YF, Tai DI, Chu CM, Chen TJ. The development of cirrhosis in patients with chronic type B hepatitis: A prospective study. *Hepatology* 1988; 8:493–6.
4. Coloquhoun SD, Belle SH, Samuel D, Pruett TL, Teperman LW. Transplantation in the hepatitis B patient and current therapies to prevent recurrence. *Semin Liver Dis* 2000; 20(Suppl 1):7–12.
5. Maddrey WC. Hepatitis B: An important public health issue. *J Med Virol* 2000; 61:362–6.
6. Beasley RP. Hepatitis B virus: The major etiology of hepatocellular carcinoma. *Cancer* 1988; 61:1942–56.
7. Lucey MR, Brown KA, Everson GT, Fung JJ, Gish R, Keeffe EB, et al. Minimal criteria for placement of adults on the liver transplant waiting list: A report of a national conference organized by the American Society of Transplant Physicians and the American Association for the Study of Liver Diseases. *Liver Transpl Surg* 1997; 3:628–37.
8. United Network for Organ Sharing, Richmond, VA. Allocation of liver policy. In *United Network for Organ Donation*; 2002.
9. Kamath PS, Wiesner RH, Malinchoc M, Kremens W, Therneau TM, Kosberg CL, et al. A model to predict survival in patients with end-stage liver disease. *Hepatology* 2001; 33:464–70.
10. Wiesner RH, McDiarmid SV, Kamath PS, Edwards EB, Malinchoc M, Kremers WK, et al. MELD and PELD: Application of survival models to liver allocation. *Liver Transpl* 2001; 7:567–80.
11. Merion RM, Schaubel DE, Dykstra DM, Freeman, Port FK, Wolfe RA. The Survival benefit of liver transplantation. *Am J Tranpl* 2005; 5:307–13.
12. Todo S, Demetris AJ, Van Thiel D, Teperman L, Fung JJ, Starzl TE. Orthotopic liver transplantation for patients with hepatitis B virus-related liver disease. *Hepatology* 1991; 13(4):619–26.
13. O'Grady JG, Smith HM, Davies SE, Daniels HM, Donaldson PT, Tan KC, et al. Hepatitis B virus reinfection after orthotopic liver transplantation. Serological and clinical implications. *J Hepatol* 1992; 14(1):104–11.
14. Belle SH, Beringer KC, Murphy JB, Detre KM. The Pitt-UNOS Liver Transplant Registry. *Clin Transpl* 1992; 6:17–32.
15. Hoofnagle JH, Di Bisceglie AM, Waggoner JG, Park Y. Interferon alfa for patients with clinically apparent cirrhosis due to chronic hepatitis B. *Gastroenterology* 1993; 104:1116–21.
16. Perrillo R, Tamburro C, Regenstein F, Balart L, Bodenheimer H, Silva M, et al. Low-dose, titratable interferon alfa in decompensated liver disease caused by chronic infection with hepatitis B virus. *Gastroenterology* 1995; 109:908–16.
17. Rosenberg PM, Dienstag J. Therapy with nucleoside analogues for hepatitis B virus infection. *Clin Liver Dis* 1999; 3:349.
18. Villeneuve JP, Condreay LD, Willems B, et al. Lamivudine treatment for decompensated cirrhosis resulting from chronic hepatitis B. *Hepatology* 2000; 31:207–10.
19. Yao FY, Terrault NA, Freise C, Maslow L, Bass NM, et al. Lamivudine treatment is beneficial in patients with severely decompensated cirrhosis and actively repli-

cating hepatitis B virus infection awaiting liver transplantation: A comparative study using matched, untreated cohort. *Hepatology* 2001; 34:411–6.

20. Perrillo RP, Wright T, Rakela J, Levy G, Schiff E, Gish R, et al. A multicenter United States–Canadian trial to assess lamivudine monotherapy before and after liver transplantation for chronic hepatitis B. *Hepatology* 2001; 33(2):424–32.

21. Fontana RJ, Keefe EB, Carey W, Fried M, Reddy R, Kowdley KV, et al. Effect of lamivudine treatment on survival of 309 North American patients awaiting liver transplantation for chronic hepatitis B. *Liver Transpl* 2002; 8(5):433–9.

22. Fontana RJ, Hann HW, Perrillo RP, Vierling JM, Wright T, Rakela J, et al. Determinants of early mortality in patients with decompensated chronic hepatitis B treated with antiviral therapy. *Gastroenterology* 2002; 123(3):719–27.

23. Yao FY, Bass NM. Lamivudine treatment in patients with severely decompensated cirrhosis due to replicating hepatitis B infection. *J Hepatol* 2000; 33(2):301–7.

24. Kapoor D, Guptan RC, Wakil SM, Kazim SN, Kaul R, Agarwal SR, et al. Beneficial effects of lamivudine in hepatitis B virus-related decompensated cirrhosis. *J Hepatol* 2000; 33(2):308–12.

25. Hann H-WL, Fontana RJ, Wright T, Everson GT, Schiff ER, Riely C, et al. Lamivudine treatment for decompensated cirrhosis due to hepatitis B: A multicenter longitudinal study (abstract). *Gastroenterology* 2001; 118:A1004.

26. Liaw YF, Sung JJY, Chow WC, et al. Impact of lamivudine on liver complications of advanced chronic hepatitis B: Results of a prospective placebo-controlled clinical trial. *N Engl J Med* 2004; 351:1521–31.

27. Leung NW, Lai CL, Chang TT, Guan R, Lee CM, Ng KY, et al. Extended lamivudine treatment in patients with chronic hepatitis B enhances HBe seroconversion rates: Results after 3 years of therapy. *Hepatology* 2001; 119:172–80.

28. Liaw YF, Leung NW, Chang TT, Guan R, Tai DI, Ng KY, et al. Effects of extended lamivudine therapy in Asian patients with chronic hepatitis B. *Gastroenterology* 2000; 119:172–80.

29. Ogata N, Fujii K, Takigawa S, Nomato M, Ichida T, Asakura H. Novel patterns of amino acid mutations in the hepatitis B virus polymerase in association with resistance to lamivudine therapy in Japanese patients with chronic hepatitis B. *J Med Virol* 1999; 59:270–6.

30. de Man RA, Bartholomeusz A, Niesters HGM, Zondervan PE, Locarnini SA. The sequential occurrence of viral mutations in a liver transplant recipient reinfected with hepatitis B: Hepatitis B immune globulin escape, famcicovir non-response, followed by lamivudine resistance resulting in graft loss. *J Hepatol* 1998; 29: 669–75.

31. Kwekkeboom J, Tha-In T, Tra WMW, Hop W, Boor PPC, Mancham S, Zondervan PE, Vossen ACTM, Kusters JG, de Man RA, Metselaar HJ. Hepatitis B immunoglobulins inhibit dendritic cells and T cells and protect against acute rejection after liver transplantation. *Am J Transpl* 2005; 5(10):2393–402.

32. Yu Z, Lennon VA. Mechanism of intravenous immune globulin in antibody mediated autoimmune disease. *N Engl J Med* 1999; 340:227–8.

33. Farges O, Saliba F, Fahramant H, Samuel D, Bismuth A, Bismuth H. Incidence of acute and chronic rejection after liver transplantation as a function of the primary disease: Possible influence of alcohol and polyclonal immunoglobulins. *Hepatology* 1996; 23:240–8.

34. Terrault NA, Zhou S, Combs C, Hahn JA, Lake JR, Roberts JP, Ascher NL, et al. Prophylaxis in liver transplant recipients using a fixed dosing schedule of hepatitis B immune globulin. *Hepatology* 1996; 24:1327–33.

35. Shouval D, Samuel D. Hepatitis B immune globulin to prevent hepatitis B virus graft reinfection following liver transplantation: A concise review. *Hepatology* 2000; 32:1189–95.

36. Celis E, Abraham KG, Miller RW. Modulation of the immunological response to hepatitis B virus antibodies. *Hepatology* 1987; 7:763–9.

37. Pruett T. Indefinite passive immunization after liver transplantation for hepatitis B. *Liver Transpl* 2002; 8(10 Suppl 1):S88–S89.

38. Samuel D. Management of hepatitis B in liver transplantation patients. *Semin Liver Dis* 2004; 24(Suppl 1):55–62.

39. Samuel D, Muller R, Alexander G, Fassati L, Ducot B, Benhamou JP, et al. Liver transplantation in European patients with the hepatitis B surface anigen. *N Engl J Med* 1993; 329(25):1842–7.

40. Samuel D, Bismuth A, Mathieu D, et al. Passive immunoprophylaxis after liver transplantation in HBsAg-positive patients. *Lancet* 1991; 337:813–5.

41. Roche B, Feray C, Gigou M, Roque-Alfonso AM, Arulnaden JL, Delvart V, et al. HBV DNA persistence 10 years after liver transplantation despite successful anti-HBS passive immunoprophylaxis. *Hepatology* 2003; 38(1):86–95.

42. McGory RW, Ishitani MB, Oliveira WM, Stevenson WC, McCullough CS, Dickson RC, et al. Improved outcome of orthotopic liver transplantation for chronic hepatitis B cirrhosis with aggressive passive immunization. *Transplantation* 1996; 61(9):1358–64.

43. Gugenheim J, Crafa F, Fabiani P, et al. Recidive du virus de l'hepatite B après transplantation hepatique. *Gastroenterol Clin Biol* 1992; 16:430–3.

44. Sawyer RG, McGory RW, Gaffey MJ, McCullough CC, Shephard BL, Houlgrave CW, et al. Improved clinical outcomes with liver transplantation for hepatitis B-induced chronic liver failure using passive immunization. *Ann Surg* 1998; 227(6):841–50.

45. Grellier L, Mutimer D, Ahmed M, Brown D, Burroughs AK, Rolles K, et al. Lamivudine prophylaxis against reinfection in liver transplantation for hepatitis B cirrhosis. *Lancet* 1996; 348:1212–5.

46. Mutimer D, Dusheiko G, Barrett C, Grellier L, Ahmed M, Anschuetz G, et al. Lamivudine without HBIG for prevention of graft reinfection by hepatitis B: Long-term follow-up. *Transplantation* 2000; 70(5):809–15.

47. Malkan G, Cattral MS, Humar A, Al Asghar H, Greig PD, Hemming AW, et al. Lamivudine for hepatitis B in liver transplantation: A single center experience. *Transplantation* 2000; 69(7):1403–7.

48. Lo CH, Cheung ST, Lai CL, Liu CL, Ng IO, Yuen MF, et al. Liver transplantation in Asian patients with chronic hepatitis B using lamivudine prophylaxis. *Ann Surg* 2001; 233(2):276–81.

49. Han SH, Ofman J, Holt C, King K, Kunder G, Chen P, et al. An efficacy and cost-effectiveness analysis of combination hepatitis B immune globulin and lamivudine to prevent recurrent hepatitis B after orthotopic liver transplantation compared with hepatitis B immune globulin monotherapy. *Liver Transpl* 2000; 6(6):741–8.

50. Marzano A, Salizzoni M, Debernardi-Venon W, Smedile A, Franchello A, Ciancio A, et al. Prevention of hepatitis B recurrence after liver transplantation in cirrhotic patients treated with lamivudine and passive immunoprophylaxis. *J Hepatol* 2001; 34(6):903–10.

51. Angus PW, McCaughan GW, Gane EJ, Crawford DH, Harley H. Combination low-dose hepatitis B immune globulin and lamivudine therapy provides effective prophylaxis against posttransplantation hepatitis B. *Liver Transpl* 2000; 6(4): 429–33.

52. Markowitz JS, Martin P, Conrad AJ, Markmann JF, Seu P, Yersiz H, et al. Prophylaxis against hepatitis B recurrence following liver transplantation using combination lamivudine and hepatitis B immune globulin. *Hepatology* 1998; 28(2):585–9.

53. Seehofer D, Rayes N, Naumann U, Neuhaus R, Muller AR, Tullius SG, et al. Preoperative antiviral treatment and postoperative prophylaxis in HBV-DNA positive patients undergoing liver transplantation. *Transplantation* 2001; 72(8):1381–5.

54. Rosenau J, Bahr MJ, Tillmann HL, Trautwein C, Klempnauer J, Manns MP, et al. Lamivudine and low-dose hepatitis B immune globulin for prophylaxis of hepatitis B reinfection after liver transplantation: Possible role of mutations in the YMDD motif prior to transplantation as a risk factor for reinfection. *J Hepatol* 2001; 34(6):895–902.

55. Yao FY, Osorio RW, Roberts JP, Poordad FF, Briceno MN, Garcia-Kennedy R, et al. Intramuscular hepatitis B immune globulin in combination with lamivudine for prophylaxis against hepatitis B recurrence after liver transplantation. *Liver Transpl Surg* 1999; 5(6):491–6.

56. Yoshida EM, Erb SR, Partovi N, Scudamore CH, Chung SW, Frighetto L, et al. Liver transplantation for chronic hepatitis B infection with the use of combination lamivudine and low-dose hepatitis B immune globulin. *Liver Transpl Surg* 1999; 5(6):520–5.

57. McCaughan GW, Spencer J, Koorey D, Bowden S, Bartholomeusz A, Littlejohn M, et al. Lamivudine therapy in patients undergoing liver transplantation for hepatitis B precore mutant-associated infection: High resistance rates in treatment of recurrence but universal prevention if used as prophylaxis with very low dose hepatitis B immune globulin. *Liver Transpl Surg* 1999; 5(6):512–9.

58. Lilly L, Girgrah N, Grant D, Mcgilvray I, Greig P, Cattrall M, Adcock L, Levy G. Successful prevention of recurrent HBV following liver transplantation using short-term low-dose HBIg in combination with lamivudine. Program and abstracts of American Transplant Congress; May 21–25, 2005; Seattle. Abstract 85.

59. Mutimer D, Pillay D, Dragon E, Tang H, Ahmed M, O'Donnell K, et al. High pretreatment serum hepatitis B virus titer predicts failure of lamivudine prophylaxis and graft re-infection after liver transplantation. *J Hepatol* 1999; 30:715–21.

60. Mutimer D, Pillay D, Shields P, Cane P, Ratcliffe D, Martin B, et al. Outcome of lamivudine resistant hepatitis B virus infection in the liver transplant recipient. *Gut* 2000; 46:107–13.

61. Xiong K, Flores C, Yang H, Toole JJ, Gibbs CS. Mutations in hepatitis B DNA polymerase associated with resistance to lamivudine do not confer resistance to adefovir *in vitro Hepatology* 1998; 28:1669–73.

62. Perrillo R, Schiff E, Yoshida E, et al. Adefovir dipivoxil for the treatment of lamivudine-resistant hepatitis B mutants. *Hepatology* 2000; 32:129–34.

63. Lok AS, Fung SK, Han SH, et al. Virological response and resistance to adefovir (ADV) therapy in liver transplant (OLT) patients. Program and abstracts of the 56th Annual Meeting of the American Association for the Study of Liver Diseases; November 11–15, 2005; San Francisco. Abstract 91.

64. Schiff ER, Lai CL, Hadziyannis S, Neuhaus P, Terrault N, Colombo M, et al. Adefovir dipivoxil therapy for lamivudine-resistant hepatitis B in pre- and post-liver transplantation patients. *Hepatology* 2003; 38:1419–27.

65. Perrillo R, Hann HW, Mutimer D, Willems B, Leung N, Lee WM, et al. Adefovir dipivoxil added to ongoing lamivudine in chronic hepatitis B with YMDD mutant hepatitis B virus. *Gastroenterology* 2004; 126:81–90.

66. Lo ML, Liu CL, Lau G, Chan SC, Ng I, Fan ST. Liver transplantation for chronic hepatitis B with lamivudine-resistant YMDD mutant using add-on adefovir dipivoxil plus lamivudine. *Liver Transpl* 2005; 11(7):807–13.

67. Hannon H, Bagnis CI, Benhamou Y, et al. The renal tolerance of low-dose adefovir dipivoxil by lamivudine-resistant persons co-infected with hepatitis B and HIV. *Nephrol Dial Transpl* 2004; 19:386–90.

68. Yang H, Westland CE, Delaney WE 4th, Heathcote EJ, Ho V, Fry J, et al. Resistance surveillance in chronic hepatitis B patients treated with adefovir dipivoxil for up to 60 weeks. *Hepatology* 2002; 36:464–73.

69. Westland CE, Yang H, Delaney WE 4th, Gibbs CS, Miller MD, Wulfsohn M, et al. Week 48 resistance surveillance in two phase 3 clinical studies of adefovir dipivoxil for chronic hepatitis B. *Hepatology* 2003; 38:96–103.

70. Dodson F, de Vera ME, Bonham CA, Geller DA, Rakela J, Fung JJ. Lamivudine after hepatitis B immune globulin is effective in preventing hepatitis B recurrence after liver transplantation. *Liver Transpl* 2000; 66:434–9.

71. Naoumov NV, Lopes AR, Burra P, Caccamo L, Iemmolo RM, de Man RA, et al. Randomised trial of lamivudine versus hepatitis B immunoglobulin for long-term prophylaxis of hepatitis B recurrence after liver transplantation. *J Hepatol* 2001; 34:888–94.

72. Buti M, Mas A, Prieto M, Casafont F, Gonzalez A, Miras M, et al. A randomized study comparing lamivudine monotherapy after short course of hepatitis B immune globulin (HBIg) in the prevention of hepatitis B virus recurrence after liver transplantation. *J Hepatol* 2003; 38:811–7.

73. Terrault NA, Wright TL, Roberts JP, Ascher NL. Combined short-term hepatitis B immunoglobulin and long-term lamivudine versus hepatitis B immunoglobulin monotherapy as hepatitis B virus prophylaxis in liver transplant recipients. *Hepatology* 1998; 28:389A.

74. Szmuness W, Stevens CE, Harley EJ, Zang EA, Alter HJ, Taylor PE, De Vera A, et al. Hepatitis B vaccine in medical staff of dialysis units. Efficacy and subtype cross-protection. *N Engl J Med* 1982; 307:1482–6.

75. Hadler SC, Francis DP, Maynard JE, Thomson SE, Judson FN, Eckemberg DF, Ostrow DG, et al. Long-term immunogenecity and efficacy of hepatitis B vaccine in homosexual men. *N Engl J Med* 1986; 315:209–14.

76. Margolis HS. Prevention of acute and chronic liver disease through immunization. Hepatitis B and beyond. *J Infect Dis* 1993; 168:9–14.

77. Keeffe EB. Vaccination against hepatitis A and B in chronic liver disease. *Viral Hepatitis Rev* 1999; 5:77–88.

78. Loinaz C, de Juanes JR, Gonzales EM, Lopez A, Lumbreras C, Gomez R, Gonzales-Pinto I, et al. Hepatic B vaccination results in 140 liver transplant recipients. *Hepatogastroenterology* 1997; 44:135–138.

79. Arslan M, Wiesner RH, Sievers C, Egan K, Zein NN. Double-dose accelerated hepatitis B vaccine in patients with end-stage liver disease. *Liver Transpl* 2001; 7:314–20.

80. Wiedmann M, Liebert UG, Oesen U, Porst H, Wiese M, Schroeder S, Halm U, et al. Decreased immunogenecity of recombinant hepatitis B vaccine in chronic hepatitis C. *Hepatology* 2000; 31:230–4.

81. Sanchez-Fueyo A, Rimola A, Grande L, Costa J, Mas A, Navasa M, et al. Hepatitis B immunoglobulin discontinuation followed by hepatitis B virus vaccination: A new strategy in the prophylaxis of hepatitis B virus recurrence after liver transplantation. *Hepatology* 2000; 31(2):496–501.

82. Sanchez-Fueyo A, Martinez-Bauer E, Rimola A. Hepatitis B vaccination after liver transplantation (letter). *Hepatology* 2002; 36:257–8.

83. Bienzle U, Gunther M, Neuhaus R, Neuhaus P, et al. Successful hepatitis B vaccination in patients who underwent transplantation for hepatitis B-related cirrhosis: Preliminary results. *Liver Transpl* 2002; 8:562–4.

84. Angelico M, Di Paolo D, Trinito MO, Petrolati A, Araco A, Zassa S, et al. Failure of reinforced triple course of hepatitis B vaccination in patients transplanted for HBV-related cirrhosis. *Hepatology* 2002; 35:176–81.

85. Starkel P, Stoffel M, Lerut J, Horsmans Y. Response to an experimental HBV vaccine permits withdrawal of HBIg prophylaxis in fulminant and selected chronic HBV-infected liver graft recipients. *Liver Transpl* 2005; 11(10):1228–34.

86. Dickson RC, Everhart JE, Lake JR, et al. Transmission of hepatitis B by livers from donors positive for antibody to hepatitis core antigen. The National Institute of Diabetes and Digestive Kidney Diseases Liver Transplantation Database. *Gastroenterology* 1997; 113:1668–74.

87. Lee KH, Wai CT, Lim SG, et al. Risk for de novo hepatitis B from antibody to hepatitis B core antigen-positive donors in liver transplantation in Singapore. *Liver Transpl* 2001; 7:469–70.

88. Uemoto S, Sugiyama K, Marusawa H, et al. Transmission of hepatitis B virus from hepatitis B core antibody-positive donors in living-related liver transplants. *Transplantation* 1995; 59:230–4.

89. Roque-Afonso AM, Feray C, Samuel D, et al. Antibodies to hepatitis B surface antigen prevent viral reactivation in recipients of liver grafts from anti-HBc positive donors. *Gut* 2002; 50:95–9.

90. Yu AS, Vierling JM, Colquhoun SD, et al. Transmission of hepatitis B infection from hepatitis B core antibody-positive liver allografts is prevented by lamivudine therapy. *Liver Transpl* 2001; 7:513–7.

91. Lee KW, Lee DS, Lee HH, et al. Prevention of de novo hepatitis B infection for HcAb-positive donors in living donor liver transplantation. *Transpl Proc* 2004; 36:2311–2.

92. Kim WR, Poterucha JJ, Kremers WK, Ishitani MB, Dickson ER. Outcome of liver transplantation for hepatitis B in the United States. *Liver Transpl* 10:968–74.

93. Gane EJ, McCaughan G, Crawford D, et al. Combination lamivudine plus low-dose intramuscular hepatitis B immunoglobulin prevents recurrent hepatitis B and may eradicate residual graft infection. *Hepatology* 2002; 36:221A.

94. de Man RA, Wolters LM, Nevens F, Chua D, Sherman M, Lai CL, et al. Safety and efficacy of oral entecavir given for 28 days in patients with chronic hepatitis B virus infection. *Hepatology* 2001; 34(3):578–82.

95. Wolters LM, Hansen BE, Niesters HG, Dehertogh D, de Man RA. Viral dynamics during and after entecavir therapy in patients with chronic hepatitis B. *J Hepatol* 2002; 37(1):137–44.

96. Kuo A, Dienstag JL, Chung RT. Tenofovir disoproxil fumarate for the treatment of lamivudine-resistant hepatitis B. *Clin Gastroenterol Hepatol* 2004; 2(3):266–72.

97. Van Bommel F, Schernick A, Hopf U, Berg T. Tenofovir disoproxil fumarate exhibits strong antiviral effect in a patient with lamivudine-resistant severe hepatitis B reactivation. *Gastroenterology* 2003; 124(2):586–7.

98. Bruno R, Sacchi P, Zocchetti C, Ciappina V, Puoti M, Filice G. Rapid hepatitis B virus DNA decay in co-infected HIV-hepatitis B virus "e-minus" patients with YMDD mutations after 4 weeks of tenofovir therapy. *AIDS* 2003; 17(5):783–4.

99. Prakoso E, Strasser SI, Koorey D, Verran D, McCaughan GW. Long-term lamivudine monotherapy prevents development of hepatitis B virus infection in hepatitis B surface antigen-negative liver transplant recipients from hepatitis B core-positive donors.

10 Liver Transplantation for Nonalcoholic Fatty Liver Disease

Michael Charlton, MD

CONTENTS

Abstract

Nonalcoholic fatty liver disease (NAFLD) is spectrum of histological findings ranging from steatosis to nonalcoholic steato-hepatitis (NASH) with progressive fibrosis and liver failure. NAFLD affects up to 30 million people in the United States with more than 600,000 with cirrhosis. With the increasing prevalence of obesity and type 2 diabetes in North America, NAFLD has become an important emerging public health issue. As the prevalence and severity of obesity continue to increase in the United States, with concomitant rises in the prevalence of type 2 diabetes and dyslipidemia, the prevalence of all grades of NAFLD can also be expected to increase. In particular, NAFLD will likely become a predominant indication for liver

From: *Clinical Gastroenterology: Liver Transplantation: Challenging Controversies and Topics*
Edited by: G. T. Everson and J. F. Trotter, DOI: 10.1007/978-1-60327-028-1_10,
© Humana Press, Totowa, NJ

transplantation in the United States over the next decade. This review describes the prevalence, clinical characteristics, and pathogenesis of NAFLD. In addition, the management of NAFLD before and after liver transplantation is discussed.

Key Words: Non-alcoholic fatty liver disease; Non-alcoholic steatohepatitis; Obesity; Diabetes; Liver transplantation

INTRODUCTION

The term "nonalcoholic fatty liver disease" (NAFLD) is used to describe a spectrum of histological findings ranging from simple steatosis to nonalcoholic steatohepatitis (NASH) with progressive fibrosis and liver failure. Based on the current prevalences of obesity and type 2 diabetes, nonalcoholic fatty liver disease can be estimated to affect between 6 and 30 million people in the United States, including over 600,000 with cirrhosis (1, 2). With epidemics of obesity and type 2 diabetes in North America, NAFLD has become an important emerging public health issue. As the prevalence and severity of obesity continue to increase in the United States (3–6), with concomitant rises in the prevalence of type 2 diabetes and dyslipidemia, the prevalence of all grades of NAFLD can also be expected to increase.

NASH is characterized by histopathological features similar to those associated with alcohol-induced liver injury, in the absence of excessive alcohol ingestion (7). The histological characteristics of NASH are macrovesicular steatosis, nuclear glycogenation, lobular and portal inflammation, and, occasionally, Mallory's hyaline (7, 8). NASH is almost always a chronic condition and is most frequently associated with obesity (central, as measured by waist circumference, and overall, as measured by BMI) and type 2 diabetes mellitus (7, 9–15). NASH can be a severe, progressive form of liver disease, leading to the development of cirrhosis (12, 13). The overall prevalence of NASH in adults in North America, based on large autopsy-based analysis, has been reported to be 18.5% in obese and 2.7% in nonobese individuals (12). Of obese individuals found to have NASH at autopsy, of which most cases were not suspected antemortem, 13.8% had bridging fibrosis or cirrhosis. The corresponding figure for lean individuals was 6.6% (12). A more recent study of the clinicopathological features of 32 patients with NASH found the prevalence of cirrhosis to be 8% (14).

CLINICAL FEATURES AND DIAGNOSIS OF NASH

Most patients who are ultimately diagnosed as having NASH are referred for evaluation of abnormal liver biochemistries, often detected serendipitously. In contrast to the ratio seen in alcoholic liver disease, aminotransferases are typically increased four or more times what is normal with ALT usually greater than AST (11, 13, 16). Alkaline phosphatase is usually elevated two or more times normal with bilirubin levels usually within the normal range (11, 13, 16).

In patients with abnormal liver biochemistries, a detailed history is essential in order to exclude, or otherwise rule out, the presence of excessive alcohol consumption, steatohepatitis inducing pharmacotherapy, surgical procedures, and occupational exposure to hepatotoxins. A nutritional history, particularly of rapid weight gain or loss, is also important. The great majority of the clinical conditions that are associated with the development of steatohepatitis can readily be excluded once a thorough history has been elicited. Of those clinical conditions associated with NASH that cannot be excluded by simple history taking, Wilson's disease, viral hepatitis, and autoimmune liver disease require serological/biochemical exclusion. The great majority of patients with NAFLD will, concomitantly, have one or more features of the metabolic syndrome (increased waist circumference, hypertriglyceridemia, low HDL cholesterol, hypertension, and a fasting glucose of 110 mg/dL or higher) (17–21).

On direct questioning, a minority of patients with NASH describe excessive fatigue and/or right upper quadrant pain (22). It is not clear whether these symptoms are more common among patients with NASH than among age-, gender-, and body mass index-matched individuals without NASH.

An ultrasonagraphic examination of the liver will detect hepatic steatosis with a sensitivity of between 66–100% (23–25), although the sensitivity is reduced for degrees of steatosis <30%. The same may be said of computed tomography, magnetic resonance imaging, and radionucleotide techniques, all of which have findings that are characteristic of hepatic steatosis. However, none of these techniques is able to distinguish simple steatosis from steatohepatitis with progressive fibrosis. As NASH is by definition a clinicohistological entity, histology is required to confirm the diagnosis.

PATHOGENESIS OF NAFLD

Although many conditions can be associated with steatosis and/or steatohepatitis, the terms "NAFLD" and "NASH" almost always refer to steatosis and steatohepatitis associated with obesity and insulin resistance/hyperinsulinemia, respectively.

It has been proposed that progression from simple steatosis to steato-hepatitis and to advanced fibrosis results from two physiological events ("hits") (26). The first event is thought to be insulin resistance, leading to the accumulation of fat within hepatocytes and associated increased lipid peroxidation. Second, the oxidative stress increases, precipitating cytokine release and, ultimately, Fas ligand-mediated hepatocellular injury.

Lipid Metabolism in NAFLD

The net accumulation of fat within hepatocytes, a prerequisite for NAFLD in general, could potentially result from alterations in the uptake, synthesis, degradation, or secretory pathways of hepatic lipid metabolism. The rate of appearance of fatty acids within hepatocytes can increase through increased

1. hepatocyte free fatty acid (FFA) synthesis,
2. uptake of circulating FFAs derived from peripheral fat stores,
3. extraction of FFAs through hydrolysis of chylomicrons via increased lipoprotein lipase activity.

Esterification of FFAs with glycerol-3-phospate, to form triglycerides and phospholipids, occurs in the presence of insulin and glucose. The rate of hydrolysis of triglycerides increases as insulin levels fall. Hyperinsulinemia, which occurs in insulin resistance, is, in contrast, associated with increased triglyceride formation and diminished rates of hydrolysis, both peripherally and within the liver. Furthermore, apolipoprotein B-100, a rate-determining step in triglyceride and FFA export from hepatocytes, is also diminished by hyperinsulinemia and in patients with NASH (27).

Obesity, when associated with hyperinsulinemia and insulin resistance, is associated with a number of metabolic effects relevant to the development of hepatic steatosis. These include increased absolute hepatic FFA uptake, increased esterification of hepatic FFAs to form triglycerides (TGs), increased FFA synthesis from cytosolic substrates, decreased apoB-100 synthesis with subsequent decreased export of FFAs and TGs, decreased hydrolysis of TGs, diminished hepatic triglyceride and FFA export, and increased beta oxidation of mitochondrial long-chain fatty acids. Although the relative contribution of these effects to the net retention of fat within hepatocytes is not known, each of the described potential contributing mechanisms to hepatic steatosis might be predicted to occur secondary to insulin resistance/hyperinsulinemia.

Insulin Resistance in NAFLD

The conditions most commonly associated with NAFLD—obesity, type 2 diabetes, and the metabolic syndrome—are heterogenic, multifactorial diseases. Based on the Third National Health and Nutrition Examination Survey (NHANES III), the overall prevalence of the metabolic syndrome in adults has been estimated to range from 24% (for individuals over the age of 20 years) to 40% for people over 60 years (28).

Both genetic and environmental factors are probably important in the pathogenesis of insulin resistance in NAFLD. The contribution of genetic factors to the risk for insulin resistance and type 2 diabetes appears to be small, however (29, 30). While genetic mutations in the insulin receptor occur, they are rare (31, 32). Although many genes may contribute to an insulin-resistant phenotype, no genetic defect has been found as the basis for insulin resistance in type 2 diabetes (33).

Obesity is strongly correlated with insulin resistance (34–36), particularly when central, or truncal (37, 38). Obesity is generally associated with multiple acquired factors predisposing to insulin resistance, including sedentary lifestyle (39), high-fat diets (40), medications (e.g., thiazide diuretics) (41), and glucose toxicity (42). While the precise mechanism of truncal obesity associated insulin resistance is not known, the release of FFAs from abdominal adipocytes into the portal circulation, with the subsequent induction of hepatic insulin resistance and stimulation of glucose (35), is likely to contribute. For the great majority of patients with NAFLD, insulin resistance seems likely to be a metabolic consequence of obesity.

In addition to the metabolic effects of obesity described above, an increased abundance of several proteins, the regulation of which is unclear, has been associated with an inhibition of insulin action. These include Rad (Ras associated with diabetes) (43) and PC-1 (a membrane glycoprotein that has a role in insulin resistance) (44), which reduces insulin-stimulated tyrosine kinase activity. Tumor necrosis factor (alpha) (45), which downregulates insulin-induced phosphorylation of insulin-receptor substrate-1 and reduces the expression of the insulin-dependent glucose-transport molecule Glut4, may also be involved in NAFLD-associated insulin resistance.

It has been proposed that leptin, which has been reported to be increased in patients with NAFLD (46–48), is a source of hepatic insulin resistance in NAFLD (49). Another potentially important factor in insulin resistance in NAFLD is adiponectin (formerly called adipocyte complement-related protein of 30 kDa) (50). Adiponectin is a 30-kDa collagen-like protein related to the C1qA, B, and C components of the complement system. Expression of adiponectin is reduced in obese mice and humans, particularly in obese individuals with type 2 diabetes. Plasma triglycerides, postprandial plasma glucose levels, and insulin sensitivity have all been shown to inversely correlate with adiponectin levels (51, 52). Weight loss and treatment with thiazolidinediones increase plasma adiponectin in animals (53) and humans (54). The administration of adiponectin to obese or diabetic mice reduces food intake, tissue triglycerides, and plasma glucose levels, while it increases insulin sensitivity and muscle FFA oxidation (53, 55, 56). The recently identified peptide hormone "resistin" (named in recognition of its association with insulin resistance) may represent a link between obesity and insulin resistance (57). The administration of anti-resistin antibody reduces blood glucose levels and increases insulin sensitivity in obese mice, whereas the administration of recombinant resistin to normal mice affects both factors negatively (57).

Oxidative Stress in NAFLD

Although the links among hepatic steatosis, inflammation, and fibrosis are not well established, increased oxidative stress—a feature of both animal models of steatohepatitis (58) and humans with NAFLD (15, 59)—is likely to play an important role. A proportion of intrahepatic lipid excess occurs in the form of unsaturated free fatty acids. The presence of unsaturated FFAs will result in increased lipid peroxidation by inducible hepatic microsomal cytochromes CYP2E1 and CYP4A (60), a highly pro-oxidant process. Extensive lipid peroxidation also occurs in cytochrome P-450 2E1 knockout mice,suggesting that cytochrome P-450 4A enzymes may be the major contributor to microsomal lipid peroxidation (60). The observation that, in a genomic analysis of histologically progressive NASH, mRNA for P-450 4A is underexpressed when compared to controls with other forms of liver disease suggests that upregulation of microsomal cytochromes may be pretranscriptionally impaired, further contributing to hepatic steatosis (61).

When pro-oxidant pathways generate more reactive species than can be consumed by antioxidant pathways (e.g., via protein disulfide isomerase or GSH peroxidase), oxidative stress occurs, with a resulting accumulation of reactive oxygen species (ROS, chiefly superoxide and hydroxyl radicals plus hydrogen peroxide). ROS can produce hepatocellular injury through several mechanisms, including direct inhibition of mitochondrial respiratory chain enzymes, inactivation of glyceraldehyde-3-phosphate dehydrogenase, inhibition of membrane Na/K adenosine triphosphatase activity, inactivation of membrane sodium channels, and other oxidative protein modifications. Reactive oxygen species are potent triggers of DNA strand breakage, with subsequent activation of the nuclear enzyme poly-adenosine 5'-diphosphate ribosyl synthetase, and eventual severe energy depletion of the cells. Mitochondrial injury (as manifested by megamitochondrion) is a hallmark of NAFLD (62–64). In addition, ROS further induce lipid peroxidation, cytokine production, and Fas ligand, all of which may contribute to the hepatocellular injury and fibrosis (65, 66). Lipid peroxidation also has the potentially important effect of resulting in the production of malondialdehyde and 4-hydroxynonenal, which serve as chemoattractants for neutrophils (necroinflammation), stimulate hepatic stellate cells (fibrosis), and upregulate transforming growth factor (TGF)-β1 expression in macrophages (fibrosis) (67). Finally, ROS mediate release of TNF-α by Kupffer cells, adipose tissue, and hepatocytes (68). TNF-α increases mitochondrial permeability, impairs mitochondrial respiration, and depletes mitochondrial cytochrome c (69, 70).

Both TNF-α-induced caspase activation and hepatocyte death (apoptosis) are increased in NAFLD (71). ROS-induced Fas ligand expression by hepatocytes is thought to contribute to hepatocyte death in NAFLD (67). Oxidative stress may be exacerbated by increased mitochondrial production of ROS secondary to impaired electron flow, as occurs in obesity (65).

Increased oxidative stress usually results in increased synthesis of protective antioxidant pathways and reactive oxygen species scavengers. Recently published data may be important in this regard. In a genomic analysis of histologically progressive NASH, three genes involved in the dismutation of reactive oxygen species (catalase, glutathione peroxidase, and Cu/Zn superoxide dismutase [SOD-1]), were diminished in subjects with cirrhosis secondary to NASH (72). This suggests a possible pretranscriptional basis of increased oxidative stress in patients with histologically progressive NASH. Decreased mRNA levels for all three ROS scavengers in patients with histologically progressive NASH suggest that the basis is likely to be at the level of transcription factor activation or synthesis. Dysregulation of ROS scavenger synthesis would account for many of the observed changes that occur in NAFLD/NASH and may play a role in the differential histological effects of hepatic steatosis that are seen among patients.

FREQUENCY OF NAFLD/NASH AS A CAUSE
OF LIVER FAILURE

There are multiple reports of the progression of NASH to end-stage liver disease (73–75). The frequency of NASH as a primary cause of liver failure among patients undergoing liver transplantation at a single large North American transplant center has been reported to have increased from 2.7% to 6.8% in a five-year period (76). These prospectively collected data provide evidence that while NASH is generally a benign condition, it can be a severe, progressive form of liver disease, leading to the development of cirrhosis and liver failure in a minority of patients. As these data are based on histological examination of explanted livers, an ascertainment bias is unlikely to have accounted for the observed increase in the prevalence of NASH as an indication for liver transplantation. The introduction of the MELD scoring system for the allocation of donor livers has not favored patients with NASH and is thus also unlikely to have affected these findings.

Given the relentless increase in the prevalence and severity of obesity in North America, combined with a younger age of onset, the frequency of NAFLD as an indication for liver transplantation would be expected to continue to increase over time. Unfortunately, the UNOS database has not recorded the frequency of NAFLD/NASH as an indication for liver transplantation until recently and data capture has been sporadic. Similarly, the NIDDK Liver Transplant Database did not list NASH or fatty liver disease as a specific indication or primary cause of liver disease. There are thus no national figures to indicate the frequency of liver disease associated with NASH as an indication for liver transplantation.

The increase in the prevalence of obesity and the reported frequency of NASH as an indication for liver transplantation have important implications for the liver transplant community as a whole. Data from the Centers for Disease Control (CDC) provide worrying clues. Figure 1 shows CDC data regarding changes in the frequency of new HCV infections and the prevalence of obesity between 1982 and 2000. Between January 1, 1998, and December 30, 2003, 22,676 liver transplants were carried out in adults in the United States according to the United Network for Organ Sharing (UNOS, www.unos.org.data). If we extrapolate the published experience nationally, the number of people undergoing liver transplantation for NASH is of the order of 1.0 per million U.S. residents/year (based on 6.4% of 22,676 adult liver transplants being carried out for NASH and assuming a mean U.S. population in 1998–2003 of 280 million; http://www.census.gov/population/www/projections).

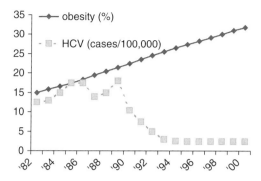

Fig. 1. CDC estimates of incidence of HCV infection and obesity in the United States, 1982–2000 (www.cdc.gov).

Based on the known increases in the prevalence of obesity in the United States (see Fig. 1) (77), the frequency of liver transplantation for NASH will increase to 2.2–4.0 cases/million U.S. residents/year in 10 to 15 years. The higher estimate reflects known increases in the severity of NAFLD with degree of obesity. Steatohepatitis is found in 3% of lean, ~20% of obese, and almost 50% of morbidly obese people (10, 12). Of severely obese patients with diabetes, 100% have at least mild steatosis, 50% have steatohepatitis, and ~20% have cirrhosis (78).

Figure 2 shows the potential impact of these changing demographics on the relative frequency of NASH as an indication for liver transplantation. Absent a safe, effective, and widely prescribed therapy for NAFLD and NASH, somewhere between 2015 and 2030, liver failure secondary to NASH will overtake HCV as the most common indication for liver transplantation in the United States. Unfortunately, in contrast

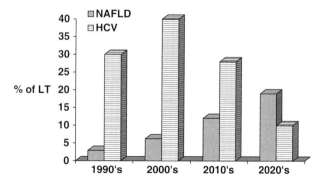

Fig. 2. Projected relative frequencies of NAFLD and HCV as indications for liver transplantation.

to the incidence of HCV, which has fallen by more than 80% from its peak, increases in the incidence and severity of obesity and NAFLD only show signs of accelerating. As NASH recurs frequently following liver transplantation and can result in graft loss (73, 79), the burden on an already stretched organ supply will be substantial. NAFLD looks set to increasingly dominate the practice of hepatology, particularly in the arena of liver transplantation. If the adipogenic and possible hepato-toxic qualities of pioglitazone, and other PPAR-γ agonists, negate their beneficial effects, we will be alarmingly short of treatment options for NASH (80). Multicenter studies aimed at identifying patients at risk for, and defining the mechanism of, progressive liver injury as well as studies aimed at optimizing the management of NASH and insulin resistance following liver transplantation are needed. The epidemic of hepatitis C infection and its impact on liver transplantation were a sur-prise. Liver failure secondary to NASH is a storm we can see a mile away.

LIVER TRANSPLANTATION FOR NAFLD/NASH

Clinical Characteristics

In the largest series reported to date, approximately half of the pa-tients evaluated for end-stage liver disease secondary to NASH were women (79). The mean age at the time of evaluation was 54.2 ± 2.8 years (range 28–70 years) and mean body mass index (BMI) was $35.5 \pm 1.8\,kg/m^2$ (range 26.1–47.2). Half of the patients evaluated for end-stage liver disease secondary to NASH had class II or III obesity (BMI > 35). One third of patients had type 2 diabetes at the time of evaluation for liver transplantation, and 38% were hypercholesterolemic and/or hypertriglyceridemic. One in six (15%) patients with end-stage liver disease secondary to NASH had undergone previous bariatric surgery (gastric stapling $n = 2$, jejunoileal bypass $n = 3$, and cardio-jejunostomy $n = 1$). One quarter of the patients undergoing liver trans-plantation for NAFLD/NASH have hepatocellular carcinoma diagnosed prior to transplantation. There is a high prevalence of MZ (17%) α_1-antitrypsin phenotypes among patients with NASH evaluated for liver transplantation. Estimates of the overall frequency of this phenotype in North America range between 2–3.6% (81–84). An association between heterozygous α_1-antitrypsin deficiency and progressive liver disease has been reported (85–88). It is possible that the combination of NASH and heterozygous α_1-antitrypsin deficiency is more likely to lead to cirrhotic stages of liver disease than NASH in isolation.

Patients with panhypopituitarism may develop NASH that is rapidly progressive, leading to cirrhosis within the second or third decade of life (89).

Outcomes Following Liver Transplantation for NAFLD/NASH

Reported one- and three-year patient survival has been 93% and 81%, respectively, following liver transplantation for NASH. Recurrence of NASH has been observed in 44% of biopsies obtained at postoperative day 7 and 60% at the fourth postoperative month. Recurrence of cirrhosis at most recent follow-up (mean 24.8, range 5.5–68.6 months) has been described in 15% of recipients, with progression to allograft failure requiring retransplantation reported in a single case. The features of steatosis may resolve histologically following the development of cirrhosis in patients with recurrence of NASH.

Treatment of NAFLD Before and After Liver Transplantation

Table 1 summarizes the published experience of treatment of NASH in humans. In lieu of a proven efficacious and safe pharmacotherapy for NASH, treatment of NASH should focus on the associated conditions. In obese patients, who make up the majority of patients with NASH, treatment should be centered around weight loss and exercise programs. Although only limited data are available, weight reduction has been shown to be efficacious in the treatment of NASH in both adults and children, as measured by aminotransferases and ultrasonographic evidence of steatosis (22, 90, 91). Attainment of an ideal body weight for height is not a prerequisite for improvement in aminotransferases and ultrasonagraphic evidence of steatosis (22, 90–92). Rapid weight loss can exacerbate steatohepatitis and hepatic encephalopathy and should be avoided (e.g., secondary to starvation diets or bariatric surgeries).

For many obese patients, sustained weight loss and exercise are, unfortunately, difficult to achieve, particularly in the setting of chronic liver disease. This has led to a proliferation of empirical and semi-empirical studies of the pharmacotherapy of NASH. Most studies of the pharmacotherapy of NASH have been small, with only a few being randomized with placebo controls. Histological follow-up is also lacking in many studies of potential treatments of NASH.

Improved glycemic control will lower lipid levels in patients with NASH who have type 2 diabetes mellitus (approximately one third of NASH patients). Glycemic control in the absence of weight loss will not, however, improve aminotransferases in this patient population

Table 1
Published Research of NASH Treatment in Humans

Treatment (Ref.)	Number of Patients	Duration of Treatment (Months)	Biochemistry	Histology
Diet + exercise (92)	31	15	Improved	n/a
UDCA (95)	24	12	Improved	Improved
UDCA + diet × 3 (101)	126	24	No change	No change
Probuchol (96)	27	6	Improved	n/a
Clofibrate (95)	16	12	No change	No change
Gemfibrozil (97)	46	1	Improved	n/a
Betaine (100)	8	12	Improved	Improved
Vitamins E and C (110)	45	6	No change	Improved
Vitamin E (98)	11	4–10	Improved	n/a
Metformin (111)	20	4	Improved	n/a
Troglitazone (112)	10	3–6	Improved	Improved
Rosiglitazone (113)	30	12	Improved	Improved
Pioglitazone and Vitamin E (80)	20	12	Improved	Improved

(93). A recent study demonstrated that metformin administration was associated with reversal of histological changes of steatohepatitis in a mouse model (94).

Metronidazole has been reported to effective in improving steatosis in patients who develop NASH following jejenuileal bypass surgery in a small, uncontrolled study (91). As jejunoileal bypass is relatively common among patients undergoing liver transplantation due to NASH, presumably due to bacterial overgrowth with translocation of lipopolysaccharide, consideration should be given to

1. Removal of atrophic, redundant loop of jejunum at time of transplantation; and
2. Long-term, suppressive antibiotics for treatment of bacterial overgrowth posttransplantation.

Very limited data are available for clofibrate (95), probuchol (a lipid-lowering agent with antioxidant properties) (96), gemfibrozil (97), vitamin E (98), n-acetyl cysteine (99), and betaine (100) in NASH. There is no conclusive evidence for a beneficial effect for any of these agents to date. Ursodeoxycholic acid treatment was associated with biochemical improvement in NASH in a pilot study (95). In a subsequent randomized, placebo-controlled study, however, ursodeoxycholic acid treatment for two years was associated with improvements in liver biochemistries and histology but at a similar frequency to that of the placebo group (101). Whether or not higher doses of ursodeoxycholic acid, as used in primary biliary cirrhosis, are effective in NASH is still the subject of study.

Based on our understanding of the pathogenesis of NAFLD/NASH, insulin sensitization is an appealing approach to treatment. An early report suggested histological and biochemical improvement in patients with NASH following therapy with a thiazolidenedione (102). Unfortunately, although pioglitazone produces histological and biochemical improvement in patients with NASH, it is associated with a significant increase in BMI as well as possible idiosyncratic hepatotoxicity (80). As PPAR-γ agonists are adipogenic by nature, weight gain is likely to be a class effect of thiazolidenediones and may well negate any histological benefit. Combined PPAR-γ/α agonists appear beneficial in animal models of steatohepatitis (103). Preliminary results of selective PPAR-α agonism in an animal model of NASH have been encouraging, with histological and biochemical improvement after short courses of PPAR-α agonism in methionine- and choline-deficient mice (104). The utility of PPAR-α agonism may be limited by the excess morbidity and mortality associated with PPAR-α agonists in large cohort studies and concerns regarding tumorigenic properties in animals (105, 106).

Choice of Immunosuppression

As discussed earlier, many patients with NAFLD have the metabolic syndrome prior to transplantation. The prevalence of dyslipidemia, hypertension, and insulin resistance increases following liver transplantation due to the effects of immunosuppression. Immunosuppression is an important factor in the development and exacerbation of posttransplant metabolic syndrome. Corticosteroids are known to produce insulin resistance, truncal fat deposition, hypertension, and dyslipidemia. Tacrolimus may be toxic to β cells. In general, calcineurin-inhibitors cause hypertension. In addition to being associated with excess death rates, infections, and hepatic artery thrombosis, sirolimus is a potent inducer of dyslipidemia. In lieu of randomized studies to determine optimal immunosuppression, steroid avoidance and minimization of calcineurin inhibition should be considered in recipients with NASH.

The Role of Protocol Liver Biopsy

The role of liver biopsy in the diagnosis and management of posttransplant NAFLD/NASH is still evolving. In addition to determining the severity of disease, a liver biopsy can also be helpful in determining the effects of medical treatment/change in immunosuppression. On the other hand, liver biopsies are associated with morbidity and cost. Several factors have been associated with a greater odds ratio of finding more severe inflammation grade and/or fibrosis stage on liver biopsy. These include age ≥ 45 years, BMI $\geq 30 \, \text{kg/m}^2$, the presence of type 2 diabetes mellitus, and a ratio of aspartate aminotransferase to alanine aminotransferase of 1 (107). Among overweight patients (BMI $\geq 25 \, \text{kg/m}^2$) with abnormal liver biochemistries, having stage 2 or higher fibrosis has been reported to be independently associated with age ≥ 50 years (odds ratio 14.1), BMI $\geq 28 \, \text{kg/m}^2$ (odds ratio 5.7), triglycerides $\geq 1.7 \, \text{mmol/L}$ (odds ratio 5), and alanine aminotransferase (ALT) $\geq 2 \, \text{N}$ (odds ratio 4.6) and independently associated with septal fibrosis. A score combining age, BMI, triglycerides, and ALT has been reported to have a 100% negative predictive value for septal fibrosis when scoring 0 or 1 (100% sensitivity for a specificity of 47%) (108). Similarly, in a small study of patients with class II obesity (BMI $\geq 35 \, \text{kg/m}^2$), the presence of two factors (out of three, including raised index of insulin resistance, systemic hypertension, and raised alanine aminotransferase) had a sensitivity of 0.8 and specificity of 0.89

for NASH (109). While of potential utility in population studies, none of the factors associated with more severe histological injury is of clear utility in the management of individual transplant recipients who may have inflammation and fibrosis despite normal transaminases. Indeed, the entire histological spectrum of NAFLD can be seen in individuals with normal ALT values, and the histological spectrum is not significantly different among patients with normal ALT from those with elevated ALT levels (19). Because NASH recurs frequently, can be severe, and cannot be predicted by biochemical profile, protocol, rather than aminotransferase-based, liver biopsies at years 1, 3, and 5 postoperatively might be considered.

REFERENCES

1. Clark JM, Diehl AM. Nonalcoholic fatty liver disease: An underrecognized cause of cryptogenic cirrhosis. *JAMA* 2003; 289:3000–4.
2. Angulo P. Nonalcoholic fatty liver disease [comment]. [Review]. *N Engl J Med* 2002; 346:1221–31.
3. Noel M, Hickner J, Ettenhofer T, Gauthier B. The high prevalence of obesity in Michigan primary care practices. An UPRNet study. Upper Peninsula Research Network. *J Fam Pract* 1998; 47:39–43.
4. Harris MI, Flegal KM, Cowie CC, Eberhardt MS, Goldstein DE, Little RR, Wiedmeyer HM, Byrd-Holt DD. Prevalence of diabetes, impaired fasting glucose, and impaired glucose tolerance in U.S. adults. The Third National Health and Nutrition Examination Survey, 1988–1994 [see comments]. *Diabetes Care* 1998; 21:518–24.
5. Popkin BM, Udry JR. Adolescent obesity increases significantly in second and third generation U.S. immigrants: The National Longitudinal Study of Adolescent Health. *J Nutr* 1998; 128:701–6.
6. Flegal KM, Carroll MD, Kuczmarski RJ, Johnson CL. Overweight and obesity in the United States: Prevalence and trends, 1960–1994. *Int J Obesity Related Metab Disorders* 1998; 22:39–47.
7. Ludwig J, Viggiano TR, McGill DB, Oh BJ. Nonalcoholic steatohepatitis: Mayo Clinic experiences with a hitherto unnamed disease. *Mayo Clin Proc* 1980; 55:434–8.
8. Lee RG. Nonalcoholic steatohepatitis: Tightening the morphological screws on a hepatic rambler. *Hepatology* 1995; 21:1742–3.
9. Samarasinghe D, Tasman-Jones C. The clinical associations with hepatic steatosis: A retrospective study. *N Zeal Med J* 1992; 105:57–8.
10. Silverman JF, O'Brien KF, Long S, Leggett N, Khazanie PG, Pories WJ, Norris HT, Caro JF. Liver pathology in morbidly obese patients with and without diabetes [see comments]. *Am J Gastroenterol* 1990; 85:1349–55.
11. Baldridge AD, Perez-Atayde AR, Graeme-Cook F, Higgins L, Lavine JE. Idiopathic steatohepatitis in childhood: A multicenter retrospective study. *J Pediatr* 1995; 127:700–4.

12. Wanless IR, Lentz JS. Fatty liver hepatitis (steatohepatitis) and obesity: An autopsy study with analysis of risk factors. *Hepatology* 1990; 12:1106–10.

13. Bacon BR, Farahvash MJ, Janney CG, Neuschwander-Tetri BA. Nonalcoholic steatohepatitis: An expanded clinical entity [see comments]. *Gastroenterology* 1994; 107:1103–9.

14. Pinto HC, Baptista A, Camilo ME, Valente A, Saragoca A, de Moura MC. Nonalcoholic steatohepatitis. Clinicopathological comparison with alcoholic hepatitis in ambulatory and hospitalized patients. *Digest Dis Sci* 1996; 41:172–9.

15. Sanyal AJ, Campbell-Sargent C, Mirshahi F, Rizzo WB, Contos MJ, Sterling RK, Luketic VA, Shiffman ML, Clore JN. Nonalcoholic steatohepatitis: Association of insulin resistance and mitochondrial abnormalities [see comments]. *Gastroenterology* 2001; 120:1183–92.

16. Powell EE, Cooksley WG, Hanson R, Searle J, Halliday JW, Powell LW. The natural history of nonalcoholic steatohepatitis: A follow-up study of 42 patients for up to 21 years. *Hepatology* 1990; 11:74–80.

17. Scheen AJ, Luyckx FH. Nonalcoholic steatohepatitis and insulin resistance: Interface between gastroenterologists and endocrinologists. *Acta Clin Belg* 2003; 58:81–91.

18. Clark JM, Brancati FL, Diehl AM. The prevalence and etiology of elevated aminotransferase levels in the United States [see comment]. *Am J Gastroenterol* 2003; 98:960–7.

19. Mofrad P, Contos MJ, Haque M, Sargeant C, Fisher RA, Luketic VA, Sterling RK, Shiffman ML, Stravitz RT, Sanyal AJ. Clinical and histologic spectrum of nonalcoholic fatty liver disease associated with normal ALT values. *Hepatology* 2003; 37:1286–92.

20. Angelico F, Del Ben M, Conti R, Francioso S, Feole K, Maccioni D, Antonini TM, Alessandri C. Non-alcoholic fatty liver syndrome: A hepatic consequence of common metabolic diseases. *J Gastroenterol Hepatol* 2003; 18:588–94.

21. Marchesini G, Bugianesi E, Forlani G, Cerrelli F, Lenzi M, Manini R, Natale S, Vanni E, Villanova N, Melchionda N, Rizzetto M. Nonalcoholic fatty liver, steatohepatitis, and the metabolic syndrome [erratum appears in *Hepatology* 2003 Aug; 38(2):536]. *Hepatology* 2003; 37:917–23.

22. Coche G, Gottrand F, Sevenet F, Ducrocq C. [Hepatic steatosis in obesity in children] [French]. *J Radiol* 1991; 72:235–7.

23. Saadeh S, Younossi ZM, Remer EM, Gramlich T, Ong JP, Hurley M, Mullen KD, Cooper JN, Sheridan MJ. The utility of radiological imaging in nonalcoholic fatty liver disease. *Gastroenterology* 2002; 123:745–50.

24. Berrut C, Curati W, de Gautard R, Widmann JJ, Godin N, Loizeau E. [The role of ultrasonography in the diagnosis of diffuse liver disease] [French]. *Schweizerische Medizinische Wochenschrift* 1986; *Journal Suisse de Medecin*, pp. 215–218.

25. Caturelli E, Squillante MM, Andriulli A, Cedrone A, Cellerino C, Pompili M, Manoja ER, Rapaccini GL. Hypoechoic lesions in the "bright liver": A reliable indicator of fatty change. A prospective study. *J Gastroenterol Hepatol* 1992; 7:469–72.

26. Day CP, James OF. Steatohepatitis: A tale of two "hits"? [Editorial]. *Gastroenterology* 1998; 114:842–5.

27. Charlton M, Sreekumar R, Rasmussen D, Lindor K, Nair KS. Apolipoprotein synthesis in nonalcoholic steatohepatitis. *Hepatology* 2002; 35:898–904.

28. Ford ES, Giles WH, Dietz WH. Prevalence of the metabolic syndrome among U.S. adults: Findings from the Third National Health and Nutrition Examination Survey. *JAMA* 2002; 287:356–9.

29. Horikawa Y, Oda N, Cox NJ, Li X, Orho-Melander M, Hara M, Hinokio Y, Lindner TH, Mashima H, Schwarz PE, Bosque-Plata L, Horikawa Y, Oda Y, Yoshiuchi I, Colilla S, Polonsky KS, Wei S, Concannon P, Iwasaki N, Schulze J, Baier LJ, Bogardus C, Groop L, Boerwinkle E, Hanis CL, Bell GI. Genetic variation in the gene encoding calpain-10 is associated with type 2 diabetes mellitus [comment] [erratum appears in *Nat Gen* 2000 Dec; 26(4):502]. *Nat Gen* 2000; 26:163–75.

30. Altshuler D, Hirschhorn JN, Klannemark M, Lindgren CM, Vohl MC, Nemesh J, Lane CR, Schaffner SF, Bolk S, Brewer C, Tuomi T, Gaudet D, Hudson TJ, Daly M, Groop L, Lander ES. The common PPAR-gamma Pro12Ala polymorphism is associated with decreased risk of type 2 diabetes. *Nat Gen* 2000; 26:76–80.

31. Saltiel AR. New perspectives into the molecular pathogenesis and treatment of type 2 diabetes [review]. *Cell* 2001; 104:517–29.

32. Kahn CR, Bruning JC, Michael MD, Kulkarni RN. Knockout mice challenge our concepts of glucose homeostasis and the pathogenesis of diabetes mellitus [review]. *J Pediatr Endocrinol Metab* 2000; 13(Suppl):84.

33. McIntyre EA, Walker M. Genetics of type 2 diabetes and insulin resistance: Knowledge from human studies [review]. *Clin Endocrinol* 2002; 57:303–11.

34. Kahn BB, Flier JS. Obesity and insulin resistance [review]. *J Clin Invest* 2000; 106:473–81.

35. Bergman RN, Ader M. Free fatty acids and pathogenesis of type 2 diabetes mellitus [review]. *Trends Endocrinol Metab* 2000; 11:351–6.

36. Boyko EJ, Fujimoto WY, Leonetti DL, Newell-Morris L. Visceral adiposity and risk of type 2 diabetes: A prospective study among Japanese Americans [comment]. *Diabetes Care* 2000; 23:465–71.

37. Banerji MA, Chaiken RL, Gordon D, Kral JG, Lebovitz HE. Does intra-abdominal adipose tissue in black men determine whether NIDDM is insulin-resistant or insulin-sensitive? *Diabetes* 1995; 44:141–6.

38. Carey DG, Jenkins AB, Campbell LV, Freund J, Chisholm DJ. Abdominal fat and insulin resistance in normal and overweight women: Direct measurements reveal a strong relationship in subjects at both low and high risk of NIDDM. *Diabetes* 1996; 45:633–8.

39. Nyholm B, Mengel A, Nielsen S, Skjaerbaek C, Moller N, Alberti KG, Schmitz O. Insulin resistance in relatives of NIDDM patients: The role of physical fitness and muscle metabolism. *Diabetologia* 1996; 39:813–22.

40. Swinburn BA. Effect of dietary lipid on insulin action. Clinical studies [review]. *Ann NY Acad Sci* 1993; 683:102–9.

41. Pandit MK, Burke J, Gustafson AB, Minocha A, Peiris AN. Drug-induced disorders of glucose tolerance [comment] [review]. *Ann Intern Med* 1993; 118: 529–39.

42. Yki-Jarvinen H. Glucose toxicity [review]. *Endocr Rev* 1992; 13:415–31.

43. Reynet C, Kahn CR. Rad: A member of the Ras family overexpressed in muscle of type II diabetic humans. *Science* 1993; 262:1441–4.

44. Maddux BA, Sbraccia P, Kumakura S, Sasson S, Youngren J, Fisher A, Spencer S, Grupe A, Henzel W, Stewart TA. Membrane glycoprotein PC-1 and insulin resistance in non-insulin-dependent diabetes mellitus [comment]. *Nature* 1995; 373:448–51.

45. Boden G. Role of fatty acids in the pathogenesis of insulin resistance and NIDDM [erratum appears in *Diabetes* 1997 Mar; 46(3):536] [review]. *Diabetes* 1997; 46:3–10.

46. Tobe K, Ogura T, Tsukamoto C, Imai A, Matsuura K, Iwasaki Y, Shimomura H, Higashi T, Tsuji T. Relationship between serum leptin and fatty liver in Japanese male adolescent university students. *Am J Gastroenterol* 1999; 94:3328–35.

47. Uygun A, Kadayifci A, Yesilova Z, Erdil A, Yaman H, Saka M, Deveci MS, Bagci S, Gulsen M, Karaeren N, Dagalp K. Serum leptin levels in patients with nonalcoholic steatohepatitis [comment]. *Am J Gastroenterol* 2000; 95:3584–9.

48. Chitturi S, Farrell G, Frost L, Kriketos A, Lin R, Fung C, Liddle C, Samarasinghe D, George J. Serum leptin in NASH correlates with hepatic steatosis but not fibrosis: A manifestation of lipotoxicity? [erratum appears in *Hepatology* 2002 Nov; 36(5):1307]. *Hepatology* 2002; 36:403–9.

49. Yahagi N, Shimano H, Hasty AH, Matsuzaka T, Ide T, Yoshikawa T, Amemiya-Kudo M, Tomita S, Okazaki H, Tamura Y, Iizuka Y, Ohashi K, Osuga J, Harada K, Gotoda T, Nagai R, Ishibashi S, Yamada N. Absence of sterol regulatory element-binding protein-1 (SREBP-1) ameliorates fatty livers but not obesity or insulin resistance in Lep(ob)/Lep(ob) mice. *J Biol Chem* 2002; 277:19353–7.

50. Tsao TS, Lodish HF, Fruebis J. ACRP30, a new hormone controlling fat and glucose metabolism [review]. *Eur J Pharmacol* 2002; 440:213–21.

51. Hotta K, Funahashi T, Arita Y, Takahashi M, Matsuda M, Okamoto Y, Iwahashi H, Kuriyama H, Ouchi N, Maeda K, Nishida M, Kihara S, Sakai N, Nakajima T, Hasegawa K, Muraguchi M, Ohmoto Y, Nakamura T, Yamashita S, Hanafusa T, Matsuzawa Y. Plasma concentrations of a novel, adipose-specific protein, adiponectin, in type 2 diabetic patients. *Arterioscler Thromb Vasc Biol* 2000; 20:1595–9.

52. Weyer C, Funahashi T, Tanaka S, Hotta K, Matsuzawa Y, Pratley RE, Tataranni PA. Hypoadiponectinemia in obesity and type 2 diabetes: Close association with insulin resistance and hyperinsulinemia. *J Clin Endocrinol Metab* 2001; 86:1930–5.

53. Berg AH, Combs TP, Du X, Brownlee M, Scherer PE. The adipocyte-secreted protein Acrp30 enhances hepatic insulin action [comment]. *Nat Med* 2001; 7:947–53.

54. Maeda N, Takahashi M, Funahashi T, Kihara S, Nishizawa H, Kishida K, Nagaretani H, Matsuda M, Komuro R, Ouchi N, Kuriyama H, Hotta K, Nakamura T, Shimomura I, Matsuzawa Y. PPAR-gamma ligands increase expression and plasma concentrations of adiponectin, an adipose-derived protein. *Diabetes* 2001; 50:2094–9.

55. Yamauchi T, Kamon J, Waki H, Terauchi Y, Kubota N, Hara K, Mori Y, Ide T, Murakami K, Tsuboyama-Kasaoka N, Ezaki O, Akanuma Y, Gavrilova O, Vinson C, Reitman ML, Kagechika H, Shudo K, Yoda M, Nakano Y, Tobe K, Nagai R, Kimura S, Tomita M, Froguel P, Kadowaki T. The fat-derived hormone adiponectin reverses insulin resistance associated with both lipoatrophy and obesity [comment]. *Nat Med* 2001; 7:941–6.

56. Fruebis J, Tsao TS, Javorschi S, Ebbets-Reed D, Erickson MR, Yen FT, Bihain BE, Lodish HF. Proteolytic cleavage product of 30-kDa adipocyte complement-related protein increases fatty acid oxidation in muscle and causes weight loss in mice. *Proc Natl Acad Sci USA* 2001; 98:2005–10.

57. Steppan CM, Bailey ST, Bhat S, Brown EJ, Banerjee RR, Wright CM, Patel HR, Ahima RS, Lazar MA. The hormone resistin links obesity to diabetes [comment]. *Nature* 2001; 409:307–12.

58. Oliveira CP, Costa Gayotto LC, Tatai C, Della Bina BI, Janiszewski M, Lima ES, Abdalla DS, Lopasso FP, Laurindo FR, Laudanna AA. Oxidative stress in the pathogenesis of nonalcoholic fatty liver disease, in rats fed with a choline-deficient diet. *J Cell Mol Med* 2002; 6:399–406.

59. Seki S, Kitada T, Yamada T, Sakaguchi H, Nakatani K, Wakasa K. In situ detection of lipid peroxidation and oxidative DNA damage in non-alcoholic fatty liver diseases. *J Hepatol* 2002; 37:56–62.

60. Leclercq IA, Farrell GC, Field J, Bell DR, Gonzalez FJ, Robertson GR. CYP2E1 and CYP4A as microsomal catalysts of lipid peroxides in murine nonalcoholic steatohepatitis. *J Clin Invest* 2000; 105:1067–75.

61. Sreekumar R, Rosado B, Rasmussen D, Charlton M. Hepatic gene expression in histologically progressive nonalcoholic steatohepatitis. *Hepatology* 2003; 38:244–51.

62. Sanyal AJ, Campbell-Sargent C, Mirshahi F, Rizzo WB, Contos MJ, Sterling RK, Luketic VA, Shiffman ML, Clore JN. Nonalcoholic steatohepatitis: Association of insulin resistance and mitochondrial abnormalities. 2001; pp. 1183–1192.

63. Rashid A, Wu TC, Huang CC, Chen CH, Lin HZ, Yang SQ, Lee FY, Diehl AM. Mitochondrial proteins that regulate apoptosis and necrosis are induced in mouse fatty liver. *Hepatology* 1999; 29:1131–8.

64. Cortez-Pinto H, Chatham J, Chacko VP, Arnold C, Rashid A, Diehl AM. Alterations in liver ATP homeostasis in human nonalcoholic steatohepatitis: A pilot study. *JAMA* 1999; 282:1659–64.

65. Pessayre D, Mansouri A, Fromenty B. Nonalcoholic steatosis and steatohepatitis. V. Mitochondrial dysfunction in steatohepatitis [review]. *Am J Physiol— Gastrointest Liver Physiol* 2002; 282:G193–G199.

66. Robertson G, Leclercq I, Farrell GC. Nonalcoholic steatosis and steatohepatitis. II. Cytochrome P-450 enzymes and oxidative stress [review]. *Am J Physiol— Gastrointest Liver Physiol* 2001; 281:G1135–G1139.

67. Poli G. Pathogenesis of liver fibrosis: Role of oxidative stress [review]. *Mol Aspects Med* 2000; 21:49–98.

68. Crespo J, Cayon A, Fernandez-Gil P, Hernandez-Guerra M, Mayorga M, Dominguez-Diez A, Fernandez-Escalante JC, Pons-Romero F. Gene expression of tumor necrosis factor alpha and TNF-receptors, p55 and p75, in nonalcoholic steatohepatitis patients. *Hepatology* 2001; 34:1158–63.

69. Tafani M, Schneider TG, Pastorino JG, Farber JL. Cytochrome c-dependent activation of caspase-3 by tumor necrosis factor requires induction of the mitochondrial permeability transition. *Am J Pathol* 2000; 156:2111–21.

70. Pastorino JG, Simbula G, Yamamoto K, Glascott PA, Jr., Rothman RJ, Farber JL. The cytotoxicity of tumor necrosis factor depends on induction of the mitochondrial permeability transition. *J Biol Chem* 1996; 271:29792–8.

71. Feldstein AE, Canbay A, Angulo P, Taniai M, Burgart LJ, Lindor KD, Gores GJ. Hepatocyte apoptosis and Fas expression are prominent features of human nonalcoholic steatohepatitis. *Gastroenterology* 2003; 125:437–43.
72. Sreekumar R, Gonzalez-Koch A, Maor-Kendler Y, Batts K, Moreno-Luna L, Poterucha J, Burgart L, Wiesner R, Kremers W, Rosen C, Charlton MR. Early identification of recipients with progressive histologic recurrence of hepatitis C after liver transplantation. *Hepatology* 2000; 32:1125–30.
73. Kim WR, Poterucha JJ, Porayko MK, Dickson ER, Steers JL, Wiesner RH. Recurrence of nonalcoholic steatohepatitis following liver transplantation. *Transplantation* 1996; 62:1802–5.
74. Molloy RM, Komorowski R, Varma RR. Recurrent nonalcoholic steatohepatitis and cirrhosis after liver transplantation [see comments]. *Liver Transpl Surg* 1997; 3:177–8.
75. Carson K, Washington MK, Treem WR, Clavien PA, Hunt CM. Recurrence of nonalcoholic steatohepatitis in a liver transplant recipient [see comments]. *Liver Transpl Surg* 1997; 3:174–6.
76. Charlton M. Nonalcoholic fatty liver disease: A review of current understanding and future impact [review]. *Clin Gastroenterol Hepatol* 2004; 2(12):1048–58.
77. Kuczmarski RJ, Carroll MD, Flegal KM, Troiano RP. Varying body mass index cutoff points to describe overweight prevalence among U.S. adults: NHANES III (1988 to 1994). *Obesity Res* 1997; 5:542–8.
78. Silverman JF, Pories WJ, Caro JF. Liver pathology in diabetes mellitus and morbid obesity. Clinical, pathological, and biochemical considerations [review]. *Pathol Ann* 1989; 24(Pt 1): 275–302.
79. Charlton M, Kasparova P, Weston S, Lindor K, Maor-Kendler Y, Wiesner RH, Rosen CB, Batts KP. Frequency of nonalcoholic steatohepatitis as a cause of advanced liver disease. *Liver Transpl* 2001; 7:608–14.
80. Promrat K, Lutchman G, Uwaifo GI, Freedman RJ, Soza A, Heller T, Doo E, Ghany M, Premkumar A, Park Y, Liang TJ, Yanovski JA, Kleiner D, Hoofnagle J. A pilot study of pioglitazone treatment for nonalcoholic steatohepatitis. *Hepatology* 2004; 39:188–196.
81. Morse JO, Lebowitz MD, Knudson RJ, Burrows B. Relation of protease inhibitor phenotypes to obstructive lung diseases in a community. *N Engl J Med* 1977; 296:1190–4.
82. Kueppers F, Dickson ER, Summerskill WH. Alpha1-antitrypsin phenotypes in chronic active liver disease and primary biliary cirrhosis. *Mayo Clin Proc* 1976; 51:286–8.
83. Webb DR, Hyde RW, Schwartz RH, Hall WJ, Condemi JJ, Townes PL. Serum alpha 1-antitrypsin variants. Prevalence and clinical spirometry. *Am Rev Respir Dis* 1973; 108:918–25.
84. Pierce JA, Eradio B, Dew TA. Antitrypsin phenotypes in Saint-Louis. In Martin JP, ed., *L'alpha-1-antitrypsine et le systeme Pi.* 1975; INSERM: Paris, pp. 71–80. WH 400 A4563.
85. Charlton MR, Kondo M, Roberts SK, Steers JL, Krom RA, Wiesner RH. Liver transplantation for cryptogenic cirrhosis. *Liver Transpl Surg* 1997; 3:359–64.
86. Graziadei IW, Joseph JJ, Wiesner RH, Therneau TM, Batts KP, Porayko, MK. Increased risk of chronic liver failure in adults with heterozygous alpha1-antitrypsin deficiency. *Hepatology* 1998; 28:1058–63.

87. Hodges JR, Millward-Sadler GH, Barbatis C, Wright R. Heterozygous MZ alpha 1-antitrypsin deficiency in adults with chronic active hepatitis and cryptogenic cirrhosis. *N Engl J Med* 1981; 304:557–60.

88. Carlson J, Eriksson S. Chronic "cryptogenic" liver disease and malignant hepatoma in intermediate alpha 1-antitrypsin deficiency identified by a Pi Z-specific monoclonal antibody. *Scand J Gastroenterol* 1985; 20:835–42.

89. Adams LA, Feldstein A, Lindor KD, Angulo P. Nonalcoholic fatty liver disease among patients with hypothalamic and pituitary dysfunction. *Hepatology* 2004; 39(4):909–14.

90. Vajro P, Fontanella A, Perna C, Orso G, Tedesco M, De Vincenzo A. Persistent hyperaminotransferasemia resolving after weight reduction in obese children [see comments]. *J Pediatr* 1994; 125:239–41.

91. Drenick EJ, Simmons F, Murphy JF. Effect on hepatic morphology of treatment of obesity by fasting, reducing diets and small-bowel bypass. *N Engl J Med* 1970; 282:829–34.

92. Hickman IJ, Jonsson JR, Prins JB, Ash S, Purdie DM, Clouston AD, Powell EE. Modest weight loss and physical activity in overweight patients with chronic liver disease results in sustained improvements in alanine aminotransferase, fasting insulin, and quality of life. *Gut* 2004; 53:413–9.

93. Seeff LB, Zimmerman HI. In Popper H, Schaffner F, eds. *Relationship Between Pancreatic and Hepatic Disease,* 5th ed. 1976; Grune and Stratton, New York, p. 595.

94. Lin HZ, Yang SQ, Chuckaree C, Kuhajda F, Ronnet G, Diehl AM. Metformin reverses fatty liver disease in obese, leptin-deficient mice. *Nat Med* 2000; 6:998–1003.

95. Laurin J, Lindor KD, Crippin JS, Gossard A, Gores GJ, Ludwig J, Rakela J, McGill DB. Ursodeoxycholic acid or clofibrate in the treatment of non-alcohol-induced steatohepatitis: A pilot study. *Hepatology* 1996; 23:1464–1467.

96. Merat S, Malekzadeh R, Sohrabi MR, Sotoudeh M, Rakhshani N, Sohrabpour AA, Naserimoghadam S. Probucol in the treatment of non-alcoholic steatohepatitis: A double-blind randomized controlled study. *J Hepatol* 2003; 38:414–8.

97. Basaranoglu M, Acbay O, Sonsuz A. A controlled trial of gemfibrozil in the treatment of patients with nonalcoholic steatohepatitis [comment]. *J Hepatol* 1999; 31:384.

98. Lavine JE. Vitamin E treatment of nonalcoholic steatohepatitis in children: A pilot study [see comments]. *J Pediatr* 2000; 136:734–8.

99. Pamuk GE, Sonsuz A. N-acetylcysteine in the treatment of non-alcoholic steatohepatitis. *J Gastroenterol Hepatol* 2003; 18:1220–1.

100. Abdelmalek MF, Angulo P, Jorgensen RA, Sylvestre PB, Lindor KD. Betaine, a promising new agent for patients with nonalcoholic steatohepatitis: Results of a pilot study [comment]. *Am J Gastroenterol* 2001; 96:2711–7.

101. Lindor KD, Kowdley KV, Heathcote EJ, Harrison ME, Jorgensen R, Angulo P, Lymp JF, Burgart L, Colin P. Ursodeoxycholic acid for treatment of nonalcoholic steatohepatitis: Results of a randomized trial [see comment]. *Hepatology* 2004; 39:770–8.

102. Neuschwander-Tetri BA, Brunt EM, Wehmeier KR, Sponseller CA, Hampton K, Bacon BR. Interim results of a pilot study demonstrating the early effects of the PPAR-gamma ligand rosiglitazone on insulin sensitivity, aminotransferases,

hepatic steatosis and body weight in patients with non-alcoholic steatohepatitis. *J Hepatol* 2003; 38:434–40.

103. Ye JM, Iglesias MA, Watson DG, Ellis B, Wood L, Jensen PB, Sorensen RV, Larsen PJ, Cooney GJ, Wassermann K, Kraegen EW. PPAR-alpha/gamma ragaglitazar eliminates fatty liver and enhances insulin action in fat-fed rats in the absence of hepatomegaly. *Am J Physiol—Endocrinol Metab* 2003; 284:E531–E540.

104. Ip E, Farrell G, Hall P, Robertson G, Leclercq I. Administration of the potent PPAR-alpha agonist, Wy-14,643, reverses nutritional fibrosis and steatohepatitis in mice. *Hepatology* 2004; 39:1286–96.

105. Miettinen M, Turpeinen O, Karvonen MJ. A co-operative trial in the primary prevention of ischaemic heart disease using clofibrate. *Br Heart J* 1979; 42:370–1.

106. Clofibrate and niacin in coronary heart disease. *JAMA* 1975; 231:360–81.

107. Angulo P, Keach JC, Batts KP, Lindor KD. Independent predictors of liver fibrosis in patients with nonalcoholic steatohepatitis. *Hepatology* 1999; 30:1356–62.

108. Ratziu V, Giral P, Charlotte F, Bruckert E, Thibault V, Theodorou I, Khalil L, Turpin G, Opolon P, Poynard T. Liver fibrosis in overweight patients. *Gastroenterology* 2000; 118:1117–23.

109. Dixon JB, Bhathal PS, O'Brien PE. Nonalcoholic fatty liver disease: Predictors of nonalcoholic steatohepatitis and liver fibrosis in the severely obese [comment]. *Gastroenterology* 2001; 121:91–100.

110. Harrison SA, Torgerson S, Hayashi P, Ward J, Schenker S. Vitamin E and vitamin C treatment improves fibrosis in patients with nonalcoholic steatohepatitis [see comment]. *Am J Gastroenterol* 2003; 98:2485–90.

111. Marchesini G, Brizi M, Bianchi G, Tomassetti S, Zoli M, Melchionda N. Metformin in non-alcoholic steatohepatitis [see comment]. *Lancet* 2001; 358:893–4.

112. Caldwell SH, Hespenheide EE, Redick JA, Iezzoni JC, Battle EH, Sheppard BL. A pilot study of a thiazolidinedione, troglitazone, in nonalcoholic steatohepatitis [see comment]. *Am J Gastroenterol* 2001; 96:519–25.

113. Neuschwander-Tetri BA, Brunt EM, Wehmeier KR, Oliver D, Bacon BR. Improved nonalcoholic steatohepatitis after 48 weeks of treatment with the PPAR-gamma ligand rosiglitazone. *Hepatology* 2003; 38:1008–17.

INDEX